Guide to Ethical Decisions and Actions for Social Service Administrators:

A Handbook for Managerial Personnel

Charles S. Levy, a social worker for over thirty-five years, has carried a wide variety of clinical, administrative, supervisory, staff and faculty development, and managerial responsibilities in both social and educational organizations. He is the author of the widely used and applauded book *Social Work Ethics* (1976), and he served as chairman of the Task Force on Ethics of the National Association of Social Workers, which produced the Code of Ethics adopted by the Association in 1979. Dr. Levy is now teaching masters and doctoral courses for social work students in administration, community social work, values, ethics, and ideology at the Wurzweiler School of Social Work, Yeshiva University, New York.

Guide to Ethical Decisions and Actions for Social Service Administrators:

A Handbook for Managerial Personnel

Charles S. Levy

A monographic supplement to
Administration in Social Work
Volume 6, 1982

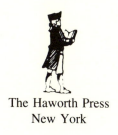

The Haworth Press
New York

© 1982 by The Haworth Press, Inc. All rights reserved. No part of this work may be reproduced or utilized in any form or by any means, electronic or mechanical, including photocopying, microfilm and recording, or by any information storage and retrieval system, without permission in writing from the publisher.

The Haworth Press, 28 East 22 Street, New York, New York 10010

Library of Congress Cataloging in Publication Data

Levy, Charles S., 1919-
   Guide to ethical decisions and actions for social service administrators.

   "A monographic supplement to Administration in social work, volume 6, 1982."
   Includes bibliographies and index.
   1. Social work administration—Moral and ethical aspects. I. Administration in social work.
Volume 6 (supplement) II. Title.
HV41.L4458   174'.9362   81-13511
ISBN 0-86656-106-4   AACR2

Printed in the United States of America

Guide to Ethical Decisions and Actions for Social Service Administrators:

A Handbook for Managerial Personnel

Contents

FOREWORD

The early 1980's are witness to a remarkable shift in national social policies and priorities. Social values and objectives achieved through fifty years of effort and conflict have seemingly been reversed, a sharp turning back of the clock. Both the rate and substance of change have been marked in the extreme. New developments in policy inevitably mandate administrative responses, and these have become increasingly apparent. The most fundamental questions of the good and the just have been raised and these are at the core questions of values and ethics.

Since many of the essential issues in the current public forum deal with social need and provision, the social and human services have become embroiled in the social marketplace. One aspect of the response has been a preoccupation with administrative-managerial questions, and with it the production of a current literature on social administration. A number of books dealing with non-profit and social service administration has appeared in the past few years, while others are in the pipeline.

Of the many aspects of the subject covered in these works and in the accompanying periodical literature, one serious omission stands out—organizational and administrative ethics. It is as though the subject and its implications were self-evident, or worse still, that their analysis was unimportant. In an area of service dealing with the human dimension, nothing could be further from the truth. In these days of diminishing resources and agonizing decisions concerning their allocation, competing values and complex ethical dilemmas increase the pressures and uncertainties which confront social administrators in all aspects of service delivery. Contradictions between the service ideal and organizational reality constitute the daily agenda of the executive who is often caught between the imperatives of organizational survival on the one hand and, on the other, the demands of honest, competent client service.

Two related phenomena have served to keep both the practice and theory of administration relatively free of moral anchoring—the pervasive American tradition of pragmatism, particularly in the politics of public administration, and Max Weber's concept of organizational man socialized into the bureaucratic mechanism of order, rationality and authority. In both strains, the canons of efficiency and utility tend to constrain ethical judgment. The very question as to whether organizations have moral rights and responsibilities (apart from what might be specified in law and legislation) pervades much current organizational thinking. Ethical neutrality is thus based upon pursuing organizational objectives through calculative rational decision-making, in which practical ends become superordinate to means and ends.

Once the organization and its controllers are perceived as moral agents, a host of dilemmas, issues and contradictions come to the surface. Professor Levy has here assayed to venture these troubled conceptual waters, and in so doing, has established a benchmark for future study and research. He deals conceptually and realistically with issues posed in considering organizational versus individual ethics, rational versus ethical models, service ideals versus empirical realities, competing organizational interests and the conflicts engendered by contradictory ethical norms. The book discusses at length the ethical relationship between administrators and the essential constituencies with which they interact, and in so doing places matters of urgency on the executive's agenda.

There has never been a time when the need for moral judgment and ethical awareness was more apparent, given the recent social policy climate and the marked diminution in resources for social purposes. Shrinking resources increase the pressures and contradictions between client service norms and organizational requirements. Scarcity enhances the influence of externalities in the organizational environment, creating sharp ethical dilemmas for executives and their colleagues pursuing service delivery objectives. When all cannot be served, who shall be denied? When organizational imperatives for survival, prestige and growth are paramount, what happens to service integrity? Should organizations have a life of their own or should they be subordinated to other purposes? While concern for efficiency and the cost-benefit calculus that accompanies it may be necessary to achieve many organizational goals, from an ethical perspective they are hardly sufficient.

Dr. Levy's book casts light on these and many other issues and questions. Its influence on the theory and practice of social administration will be important. Administrators who read and study it will be vastly enriched.

Simon Slavin

ACKNOWLEDGMENTS

When a person receives an award for achievement, say in the performing arts, and proceeds to catalogue those to whom a debt of gratitude is owed, benefactors may pay tearful attention—perhaps to make sure they have not been forgotten—but others are likely to yawn. On the other hand, to abstract one's thanks—"there are so many to whom I owe so much, so I won't mention anybody"—borders on ingratitude.

And yet, that is just about what I am moved to say, and it may be the only way I can in justice say it. Art Ford, a fellow thespian with whom, among others, I did occasional play excerpts for courageous audiences in New York City's Department of Health building during *the* Depression, and who subsequently became a prominent disc jockey, found a clever solution to a similar problem. In a two-page spread in a picture magazine appeared around his likeness a mass of miniature photographs representing all of those who had had a hand in his climb to fame. That was Art Ford's way of depicting the many people who had helped him in his career.

This is no "Oscar," or "Tony," or even an "Emmy." It is only a book, and, Lord knows, there are plenty of those these days. But in its pages are clearly reflected the debt—the debts—I owe to those upon whose wisdom I have drawn, to those who have taught me, inspired me, encouraged me, and to many others who directly or indirectly have affected me and, consequently, this book.

I need begin only with the scholars and writers whom I have cited, and others who may not be quoted but whose influence is evident in these pages. There have of course been others—friends, colleagues, associates, and family—in my experience as a businessman and as a social worker who have been important sources of insight and understanding. That adds up to a lot of people to whom I remain grateful.

But I would like to specify a few individuals whose contributions to this book should not be obscured by generalizations. There is Dr. Simon Slavin, editor of *Administration in Social Work,* for example. He invited me to write this book and provided encouragement and guidance as I undertook to do so. Miss Faye Zucker, Senior Editor of Haworth Press, did a great deal to facilitate the publication of the book. It has also been a pleasure to do business with Mr. William Cohen, publisher of Haworth Press. Miss Pearl Seidenberg helped a lot to put the manuscript in sufficient order for processing.

The National Association of Social Workers was kind enough to permit me to reproduce its Code of Ethics, the relevance of which is readily evident throughout the book.

All in all I have found this a gratifying and thought-provoking enterprise. I'm glad I did it and I'm grateful to everyone who helped.

Charles S. Levy
October 6, 1981

Guide to Ethical Decisions and Actions for Social Service Administrators:

A Handbook for Managerial Personnel

I. INTRODUCTION

Since this is a book about ethics, it is plausible for author and reader to come to terms about mutual expectations, for the mutuality of expectations is of the essence of ethics.

Ethics in General

Ethics, in effect, is a function of the relationship between parties to any transaction, and the responsibilities which inhere in that relationship. Or vice versa. This applies to the relationship between parent and child, husband and wife, employer and employee, and so on. It is certainly true of the relationship between doctor and patient, lawyer and client, and social worker and client. And it is true of the relationship between administrator and a variety of persons and institutions to whom and to which the administrator's job responsibility is in some way connected.

What This Book Is and Is Not About

As for author and reader, it seems desirable, if not necessary, to set forth the boundaries of expectation at the very beginning, especially at the beginning of a book like this. One way of doing this is to make clear what the reader has a right to expect. Another is to define limits to the reader's expectations. Both correspond to responsibilities incurred in any relationship, and particularly in a relationship in which one of the participants provides a service and the other receives that service, or performs a function which affects others. Aside from the practical considerations which dictate such an arrangement, there are also moral considerations. What is of concern is not only what will work in the implementation of responsibility, but also what is *owed* by way of responsibility. That is one of the distinguishable features of ethical responsibility.

Ethics is not a one-way street. However unilaterally ethical responsibility may be defined for a professional relationship—for example the relationship between practitioner and client, or between administrator and subordinate—to thus emphasize what one owes to the other, the latter carries a share of ethical responsibility. A minimal application of this—may we call it a principle for the moment?—a minimal application of this principle to the author-reader relationship, to the extent that it is a relationship, would require the reader to expect what the reader has been led by the author to expect, and not something else.

1

In this spirit, let me emphasize that, although this is a book about the ethics of social work administration, it is not a book about administration as such. Fortunately, enough books on administration are, and continue to be, available not to necessitate another one. They deal with such subjects as budgeting, planning, personnel, control, public relations, accounting, evaluation, etc.—all the processes and tasks required in the administration and management of organizations. Still, one can hardly expect much by way of intelligibility about the ethics of administration, whether in social or business organizations, without a foundation in the substance of administration. And therein lies the tale of this book.

What is attempted in this book is the overlaying on the subject of social work administration—the administration of social organizations—of a kind of prism of ethics. What must be avoided, however, is the construction, in the process, of a "prison" of ethics. What I mean to say is that, despite the focus on ethics, which presumably underscores the moral dimension of administration, its relevance to the practical dimensions of administrative responsibility must be constantly evident. Although the ethics of administrative practice is not measured by criteria of administrative competence, ethical practice without administrative competence borders on the fatuous. The consideration of the ethics of social work administration cannot fruitfully be divorced from the purposes and processes of social work administration. That means that though this book cannot be relied on to illuminate the substance of administrative processes and practices, it must be premised on such substance if it is to have any practical meaning and utility.

The Source of Ethics in Social Work Administration

Ethics in social work administration derives from the substance of administrative processes and practices, and from the definition of administrative responsibility. To say this is to appear to neglect G. E. Moore's caution against what he described as the naturalistic fallacy (1968). Moore considered it a fallacy to derive the "ought" from the "is," which is to say, to derive values from facts. On the face of it, Moore's caution seems to be well-taken but, as others have counseled (Klemke, 1969), it can still be taken too literally at best, and at worst it can constrict thought and opportunity unduly.

It may of course be hazardous to move too freely from facts to values, especially, as Moore suggested, when values are presumed to inhere in, and therefore flow directly from facts. This presumption must be regarded as fallacious since values do not exist as a natural consequence of facts. They do not exist at all until somebody puts them there. To say, therefore, that values may be derived from facts is not the same as saying that the values are already contained in the facts, as long as it is understood that someone or some group is actually doing the deriving—someone or some group is attaching values to facts discovered or uncovered.

The purposes, policies, procedures, and practices of organizations which are administered, along with the participants and the relationships associated with them, constitute the facts of administration to which values may be attached, or from which values may be said to be derived. Some purposes, procedures, policies, and practices may be regarded as "good"—or, more accurately perhaps, they may be adopted and employed *because* they are preferred and hence regarded as good. Others may be avoided, on the other hand, because they are not preferred or regarded as preferable or good. The judgment of preferability or "goodness" may, however, not be related at all to intrinsic worth. Rather, it may be a preference based simply on expedience, or convenience, or timeliness, or sheer bias.

Reasonable minds may certainly differ about which policies, practices, purposes, and procedures to characterize one way or another, not only in general but also under particular circumstances. Individuals and groups may therefore share values—they may agree that they prefer similar things—but differ about which they choose under different circumstances or at different times, or about the ways of attaining them. In analyzing administrative situations, one must examine both the values which guide or influence the participants in them—that is, the values which the participants carry with them into those situations—and the values which become operational in those situations because of the very nature of the situations. When the participants are associated with occupational expectations because of their membership in occupations which have codes of ethics, or because of responsibilities assigned to them which are associated with particular customs and usages, values may also be attributed to them whether or not they are manifestly guided or influenced by those values. When any of these orders of value is involved in administration and pertains to its practice, questions and considerations of ethics emerge, for ethics, as should become evident shortly, is the behavioral dimension of values.

Values, whether as abstractly conceived preferences or as preferences regarding behavior in relation to others, and particularly in the context of assigned or attributed responsibility, are chosen. They do not simply exist. If they can be said to exist, they exist as ideas which may then be applied either by way of practice or by way of expectation to particular realities and circumstances. Organizations which are administered and managed are such realities, and in them are experienced a variety of circumstances to which values are relevant, including values pertaining to the conduct of organizational participants, which is to say their ethics.

Ethics in Social Work Administration as Administrative Ethics

When one appraises what is done by the participants in these circumstances, and about these circumstances, on the basis of what is or is not valued, one enters the sphere of administrative ethics. Similarly, when one selects or prescribes what is preferable to be done in these circumstances, one has entered the realm of administrative ethics. There are other kinds of ethics as well in organizations, depending on the kinds of purposes they serve and the kinds of activities in which organizational participants engage in the implementation of those purposes—the ethics of social work practice, for example, when social work is one of the activities of the organization. But administrative ethics describes ethical responsibility and ethical practices at the level at which participants and organization relate to one another in the fulfillment of organizational purposes. When the primary activity of the organization, the activity for which the organization or a department of the organization has been primarily established, is social service of some kind, the sphere of concern will be described in this book as the ethics of social work administration.

Administrative ethics therefore represents what is valued by way of deeds or omissions in the administration of organizations—any organization—as well as what is done in the light of these preferences. Administrative ethics thus becomes a basis for judgments regarding what has already been done in that light. Such judgments may be made and, when formal provision is made for making and acting on such judgments, as in the case of disciplinary and grievance procedures, such judgments *are* made on the basis of available facts. A negative judgment signifies unethical conduct. That is, it signifies that whatever was done or not done conflicted with the values which have been selected as guides to conduct in an administrative capacity.

To recapitulate, organizations are administered by persons—variously called managers or administrators, or both—who have assigned and acknowledged responsibility to manage and administer those organizations. Organizations, having their own history and their own cultures, establish and accumulate their own conceptions of behavior preferred or expected of administrators. Such preferences and expectations are also derived from social and occupational idealizations of administrative behavior. In the occupations represented in the organizations, and in the community and society at large, ideas emerge and are often codified to guide and govern the conduct of persons with administrative responsibility. To the extent that organizations vary with respect to purposes, functions, and norms, their preferences and expectations are apt to vary. Nevertheless, there seems to be a body of values on the basis of which preferences and expectations are formulated and enunciated, which are common to all organizations—certainly in North America.

The behavioral preferences and expectations which serve as guides to administrative practice also serve as bases for evaluation. On such bases the conduct of administrators can be appraised by persons in the organizations with authority over the administrators. Boards of directors usually carry such authority in voluntary social organizations. The conduct of administrators may also be judged by persons outside of the organizations whose views and influence matter to the organizations.

Ethics Versus Competence

Not all judgments of administrative conduct are ethical judgments. Many judgments in and of organizations are judgments of competence—that is, judgments regarding the ability and capacity of administrators to do the job assigned or ascribed to them. Some abilities and capacities are valued more than others. This does not make conduct affected by such abilities and capacities ethical or unethical. However, a morality of administrative behavior may be devised or ordered to guide and govern administrative conduct, and conduct in an administrative capacity, on the basis of which ethical judgments may be made. Such judgments would relate not to how well or proficiently the administrative work is done and the administrative responsibilities are carried out, although these, too, would be influenced by preferences regarding both. They would relate rather to the values affecting the manner in which the work is done and the responsibilities carried out.

A morality of administrative behavior and conduct in an administrative capacity would constitute the ethics of administration. When administrative responsibility is carried in a social agency or organization, the morality which guides and governs conduct in the fulfillment of administrative responsibility constitutes the ethics of social work administration. That is what this book is primarily about. Particular attention, moreover, will be paid to the administration of voluntary social organizations, although much that will be said applies to governmental organizations and even to business and industrial organizations.

Morality, Morals, Ethics, and Justice Distinguished

I use the term "morality" as a generic characterization of any system of values or valued conduct. Thus, ethics represents a morality affecting relationships among persons, and professional ethics represents a morality affecting the conduct of practitioners in a given occupation. Justice, on the other hand, represents a morality affecting the rights of persons in a system either of law or social relationships. Nevertheless, ethics may be regarded as a response to the rights of individuals or groups which may be affected by the actions or omissions of others. In this sense, then, ethics is also a function of justice, or a means for insuring that justice is done.

Morality must be distinguished from morals, however. Morals represent conduct preferred or expected of persons on the basis of existing social norms, and judged accordingly. It is not so judged in relation to roles or responsibilities carried by actors. The conduct of anyone engaging in such behavior would be similarly judged, although the conduct of individuals with some roles in society—priests or judges, for example—might be more severely judged than others. Some unethical conduct might, therefore, also be considered immoral, but in its own right rather than as conduct in a professional capacity. Indecent exposure or child molestation would be adjudged immoral (legal considerations aside) no matter who did it or to whom. But if a school teacher did it to one of the pupils in a class, it would also constitute unethical conduct.

Accountability for the Ethics of Social Work Administration

The ethics of social work administration applies to all of the administrator's relationships for, to all of the persons with whom the administrator deals or whom the administrator affects in the implementation of administrative responsibility, the administrator has attributable ethical responsibility. The ethics of social work administration also applies to the myriad situations and institutions that the administrator encounters in the course of administrative practice. The very nature of the situations and of the encounters suggests the moral imperatives and expectations by which the administrator may be held to be bound. Even in the highest position in an organizational hierarchy, in which an administrator may enjoy ultimate organizational authority, an accounting is expected on ethical as well as other grounds, and an accounting must be made. In fact, it is the exalted nature of that very position which makes such an accounting a requirement.

Who expects the accounting, and to whom it is due, are matters to be considered later. However, what should be kept in mind is the fact, as well as necessity, in dealing with the ethics of social work administration, that the administrator, at any level of administrative operation, is not the sole arbiter of the ethics to be applied or the ethics to be evaluated either in general or in any particular instance. Even privately made choices of action in confrontations with issues of an ethical nature—choices of which only the administrator may be aware at the time—are subject to external scrutiny. Social organizations—especially voluntary organizations—generally have boards of directors. Administrators have colleagues, and they have professional peers inside and outside the organization. And organizations are surrounded by other organizations, institutions, and communities with a stake or interest in what the organizations do or do not do, and hence with a stake or interest in what the administrators of those organizations do or do not do. Whether or not any of these organizations, institutions, or communities ever looks into the administrator's practices, the administrator is duty-bound to take their views and responses into account. Duty is an ethical concept. And ethics is a social concept. No administrator is ever entirely alone, despite what is often described as the loneliness of the administrative job.

With so many parties sharing an interest in the administrator's ethics, especially in organizations committed to one important social purpose or another, one might assume a high degree of consensus about what is and what is not ethical conduct in an administrative capacity. But this is hardly the case. There are likely to be differences among persons—even among persons who share particular conceptions of administrative processes—regarding what is and what is not to be valued by way of administrative conduct in particular administrative situations. It is invariably a matter of choice; one might almost say that it is frequently a matter of ethical taste about which it is sometimes hard to argue. The difference in relation to administrative ethics is that transcendent norms are just as likely to exist and thus to limit the freedom of choice on the part of administrators.

The Value Base of Social Work Administration

The choice of values by which administrative behavior may be guided, and upon which criteria of evaluation may be based, can be both consensual and systematic. Despite the ostensibly nonrational character of values, whether as applied to objects, or to concepts, or to behavior (as in ethics), they can be rationally selected and rationally applied. Thus, though values are a function of arbitrary choice and hence a matter of virtual taste, they may be rationally founded. The concept of *de gustibus non disputandum est* may be a truism as far as personal tastes are concerned—like those affecting foods and fashions— but it is dysfunctional as far as administrative values and ethics are concerned. What requires careful consideration, therefore, is the context of administrative practice and the value premises which may be consensually conceded to be relevant to it as the means and requisites of ethical administrative practice. Both will be considered here. In any case, given an analysis of the context of administrative practice, and agreement regarding the values by which administrative practice is validly guided and evaluated, decisions regarding both may be rationalized, documented, and substantiated. Carried far enough, processes like these can and do lead to the codification of applicable ethics.

A code of ethics which is designed to guide and govern the moral aspects of administrative practice in effect represents a consensus among persons and institutions, with influence and a degree of authority over administrators, regarding behaviors to be preferred and encouraged in particular organizational circumstances, and behaviors which may be subject to censure and disciplinary action. A code of ethics is usually composed of principles of ethical conduct, as well as prohibitions of conduct, which can serve as guides for ethical practice in an administrative capacity, and for evaluations of practice from the point of view of ethics.

Relatively few principles of ethics in social work administration have been codified. Not all of these are universally conceded by administrators of social organizations to be valid as guides to ethical conduct or as criteria for the evaluation of administrative behavior. Differences remain among them—if not about the principles as such, then about their application or operation. Principles of ethics in social work administration have by no means been exhaustively formulated even for the purpose of testing for consensus among administrators and others concerned about administrative practice in social organizations. The focus of attention here will therefore be the value implications of what goes on in the administration of social organizations—especially voluntary social organizations—and of what, as a result, is at risk and at stake in what goes on for the organizations, for organizational participants, and for others concerned with them or affected by them.

Since administrators have a lot to do with what goes on in social organizations, they are affected by the value implications of what does go on and carry considerable responsibility in relation to them. Translated into behavioral expectations, these value implications amount to ethics. It should be of interest therefore to consider not only such principles of ethics as already exist, whether in formally adopted codes of ethics or as occupational norms, to guide and evaluate administrative conduct, but also what principles perhaps ought to exist in view of the nature and circumstances of administrative practice.

Ethics for and by People

Ethics has meaning only in relation to people. It is people who are or are not ethical. And people are the primary reason why ethics—any ethics—is necessary. Even if it may be said with considerable accuracy that administrators have ethical responsibility in relation to the organizations by which they are employed—and this may indeed be so said—it is as entities made up of human beings and for human beings that organizations must be viewed. It is as social systems with purposes and stakes for people, with significance for people, and with consequences for people, that organizations are owed ethical responsibility by their administrators. It is also as social systems that organizations owe ethical responsibility to others, but it is the people who run the organizations in whom this responsibility is lodged. Organizations cannot be ethical or unethical. Only people can be. And the leadership of organizations can formulate and adopt policies for administrative implementation which are ethical or unethical in their administrative effects.

As Harleigh B. Trecker insisted, with his own italics, *"The real focus of administration is relationships with and between people"* (1950, p. 2). Ethics is indeed a function of the relationships among persons and of the defined and implied responsibility they carry in relation to one another. The ethics of social work administration is a function of the relationships within social organizations and of the relationships between those organizations and other organizations and persons.

The Starting Point of Ethics in Social Work Administration

In an important sense, the starting point of the ethics of social work administration—as of ethics in general—is the expectation that whatever a person or group is responsible, by assignment, relationship, or attribution to do, that person or group will in fact do. Accountability for doing what is thus expected is incurred. To neglect to do that for which one is accountable is unethical since such neglect represents the failure to fulfill an assigned, ascribed, or assumed undertaking. Such an undertaking can hardly be unilaterally defined. It requires some sort of social definition, whether by contract, job description, custom and usage, or other medium of social understanding. The consent of the person who is expected to be ethical is therefore not always necessary. Whether or not a social organization administrator knows what is expected by way of ethical conduct, or even considers it valid, the expectation applies. On the other hand, the expectation must be based on reasonable grounds. For that purpose, a thorough and unbiased appreciation of the nature and circumstances of administrative practice and responsibility, and of the specific responsibilities of the administrator is essential.

Within the framework of assigned or ascribed administrative responsibility, in social organizations certainly but also in other types of organizations, a variety of situations and relationships is generated. In relation to these, some behaviors may be valued while others may not be valued. Organizational and occupational norms as well as societal norms can be resorted to for a determination of which behaviors are to be valued and which are not. As multitudinous and multifarious as these may be, however, they may be insufficient for the purpose of such a determination. For one thing, they may include too many contradictions. Some highly creditable values may be diametrically opposed to other equally creditable values, either in general or in their application to practice problems and issues. Loyalty to an organization on the part of an administrator may be valued and therefore expected, for example, and the administrator may agree completely. But the collective interest of the community of which that organization is but a part, may cause to be set off against that value the value of superseding loyalty to the community. And the administrator may agree with that, too. Some principle of ethical conduct may be needed to help the administrator cope with, and perhaps resolve that conflict. But both values do operate in such a case and neither can be cavalierly dismissed—not without some accounting to somebody, even if that somebody is only the administrator.

Organizational, occupational, and societal norms as such may also be insufficient for a determination of what is or is not to be valued in the ethical resolution of a problem in administrative practice. Despite their apparent relevance to the problem, they may not serve the purpose which may be required of ordering priorities among the various values applicable to the problem. Such priority ordering may be necessary in view of the differential ethical responsibilities owed by the administrator to various persons and institutions affected by the problem or its solution, or perhaps both.

It is also conceivable that organizational, occupational, or societal values may not have been differentiated, formulated, or enunciated, or legitimated sufficiently, if at all. They would then have to be invented or reconsidered in relation to administrative responsibility, either in general or in particular instances, in order to serve as guides or evaluative criteria for ethical administrative practice. Changes in social conditions and situations may also lead to changes in values and expectations.

To take a historically transplanted example, before governmental responsibility for income maintenance was institutionalized in the United States in 1935, thus to relate the ethics of social work responsibility to legislated policy, the ethics of the social work administrator was derived from norms of charitable giving and distribution of long standing. But some of these norms had become irrelevant, given the pervasive effects of a massive depression and the obsolete capacity of private charities. New norms of ethical practice were required, as was a period of adjustment for administrators of voluntary social organizations. The strains of the transition from one system to the other were frequently evident. Recipients of public assistance and social security could not be sure, on the basis of the way in which they were treated by administrators, that what had been a function of good will was now a matter of legal right.

A more futuristically oriented illustration, although perhaps a rather far-fetched one, might be a social service administered on a space platform beset by ethical issues affecting the administrator's relationship to clients, to managers of scientific equipment and experiments, to political leaders, to the government on the mainland of the United States, and perhaps to a neighboring space platform operated by a Soviet Union which found itself (still) in political and military conflict with the United States.

The Changing Nature of the Ethics of Social Work Administration

The ethics of social work administration, for all these reasons as well as others, is obviously subject to revision, amendment, refinement, and elaboration. Its applications are also subject to reconsideration for the same reasons. Another provocation to change in the ethics of social work administration is such modification in the conception of administrative responsibility as occurs as a result of emerging philosophies of administration, and societal changes that occasion them and have impact on them. There is little doubt that the shift from scientific management to humanistic administration, both of which have played their role in social work administration, has led to reorientations with respect to the ethics of social work administration, and has been influenced and affected by the ethics of social work administration in turn.

Size and complexity of organizations are not insignificant variables in relation to the ethics of social work administration. Large and complex organizations tend to increase the number of persons who can be affected by the ethics of social work administrators, and the number of opportunities to be affected by them. They tend also to have more administrators by whom to be affected. At the higher levels of the administrative hierarchy of large and complex organizations, moreover, greater power over more persons tends to be concentrated. This intensifies the need for ethics and for sensitivity and clarity about ethical judgments.

But size and complexity need not be the critical variables, or the variables which help to explain differences regarding orientations and practices in relation to ethics. David A. Balla's observation regarding the relationship of institution size to quality of care in institutions for retarded persons seems just as applicable to the relationship of size to ethics either as idealized or as realized:

> Size is a demographic variable, not a social or psychological one. . . . Even if size were found to be associated with quality of care, the question would remain as to what factors actually contributed to the more or less adequate care. The range of possibilities is large. . . . Even if smaller size were found to be associated with better quality of care, one could not be certain that size was the crucial variable (1976, p. 118).

Complexity as well as size is certainly not the only or even the most important factor in determining the level of ethical responsibility appropriate in an organization, or in predicting the level of ethics operative in it, although it can perpetrate its influence. Left to their own natural consequences, perhaps, the factors of size and complexity might have great influence on the ethics of social work administrators in organizations. If size and complexity are regarded as consequential for the ethics of social work administration, consideration may have to be given to compensatory influences and devices to reduce their impact in the interest of ethical administrative practice.

All of this is by way of setting the stage for the discussion of the ethics of social work administration. Before going into the discussion in any detail, it may be helpful to consider some of the concepts upon which the discussion will rely, along with the organizational context to which they are germane.

REFERENCES

Balla, David A. "Relationship of Institution Size to Quality of Care: A Review of the Literature," *American Journal of Mental Deficiency* 81 (1976), 117-124.

Klemke, E. D., ed. *Studies in the Philosophy of G. E. Moore* (Chicago: Quadrangle Books, 1969).

Moore, George Edward. *Principia Ethica* (Cambridge: The University Press, 1968). First Edition published in 1903.

Trecker, Harleigh B. *Group Process in Administration* (Enlarged ed. rev.; New York; Woman's Press, 1950).

II. CONCEPTS AND CONTEXT

The ethics of social work administration, I have said, is a function of administrative responsibility in social organizations, and of the relationships which that responsibility engenders and requires. Administrative responsibility is widely shared and widely dispersed, however. Since administrative responsibility varies in nature and significance, depending upon the status and position in an organization of those who carry that responsibility, the nature and significance of their ethical responsibility will also vary. Distinctions must therefore be made regarding who carries what responsibility, and the import it has for the ethics of social work administration.

Ethics Is Everybody's Business in Social Organizations

It may be said with considerable confidence at the very outset that no one in a social organization is altogether exempt from ethical responsibility, although ethical responsibility cannot be said to be officially assigned to everyone in the organization. The members of the board of directors of a voluntary child welfare agency, for example, are not employees; nor are they paid for their efforts. They are not engaged in a specifiable occupational role in the agency, and hence cannot be bound by the occupational norms attributed to child welfare workers and others whose vocational mission it is to serve children, their families, and foster parents. And yet, the status and position of board members in the agency, for the purpose of some kind of social control, requires of them ethical aspirations and constraints of one kind or another. The responsibilities they carry, the authority with which they are cloaked, the decisions they are authorized to make, and the effects they can have make such aspirations and constraints necessary.

The ethics of social work administration, therefore, applies in some measure to agency board members as well as agency staff members. Consideration must be given to their ethical responsibility, and to the ways in which that responsibility differs, if it does, from the ethical responsibility of paid staff members, especially staff members who have specific occupational identities or identifications—as social workers, for example. Similarly, although all agency staff members share administrative responsibility, there are differences among them with respect to the nature and extent of their ethical responsibility in the administrative context, depending upon their roles, functions, and relationships in the agency.

To provide for the wide range of effects of organizational administration, and the diversity of personnel with defined or attributable administrative responsibility, three categories of ethics may be delineated which characterize the operation and application of administrative ethics in social organizations. They also identify both the sources and levels of ethical responsibility in social organizations.

Categories of Ethics in Social Organizations

The three categories of ethics are (1) general ethics, (2) organizational ethics, and (3) occupational ethics. Each of these categories may be further subdivided into additional categories for, within each, sources and levels of ethical responsibility may be further differentiated.

General Ethics

General ethics defines the moral obligations which individuals and groups may be said to have towards others because of the nature of their relationship to them. Although not always enforceable in the society at large—not, at least, in a formal manner—these moral obligations set or reflect standards of conduct applicable to those relationships. The relationships to which the obligations apply are of common experiential vintage and not associated with the occupational roles of those to whom the obligations are attributed. To the extent that relationships in and among social organizations correspond to those social relationships to which ethical standards are regarded as applicable, to that extent those standards are attributed to intraorganizational and interorganizational relationships.

Thus, in the society at large, parents are charged with ethical responsibility toward their children. This is aside from the expectations provided for in the law, since, as valued behavior, the expectations would apply even in the absence of law. They might, for example, operate as social norms. Social sentiment assumes the existence of parental love, and hence leads to specific behavioral expectations in relation to children, despite the relative unreliability of the assumption to begin with. In addition, however, the bearing of children by parents, and the dependency of the children upon them, leads to the valuation of parental care and the expectation that such care will be made available to the children.

This may be an existential expectation, but it is also a moral judgment. The moral judgment may, in fact, be reinforced by the existential expectation. The neglect of what is an anticipated natural act is likely to be subject to more intensive moral judgment. What is assumed to exist in nature becomes an imputed moral obligation, which then becomes the basis for social pressure or disciplinary or punitive action. Moral obligations, however, need not be founded on assumptions about what exists. They may be based on an appraisal of what does exist, by way of situations and relationships, for example.

The expectation or valuation of parental care shapes expectations which are formulated as parental ethics. These expectations often become so forceful that they are legislated and made formally enforceable. Parents who fail to fulfill their ethical responsibility by neglecting the care of their children, or by injuring them, are subject to criminal penalties.[1] But under the system of social control to which they are subject, they would be held to the same expectations even if there were no laws to govern their conduct in relation to their children. The sanctions would simply be different and operate differently; and not necessarily less effectively.

A key consideration in the emergence and development of the principles of ethics to guide and evaluate the conduct of parents in relation to their children is the dependency of the children and their involuntary status as dependent children. Parents are, of course, affected in their responsiveness to their ethical responsibility by many other psychological, social, and environmental influences. But the significance of general ethics lies, not so much in what people feel moved to do because of values they are committed to and aspire to, as in what others expect them to do in light of the values to which the community or society is predominantly committed. If both coincide, all well and good. If not, it is what is expected by others that ultimately counts for the judgment to be made that what has been done is or is not ethical.

Dependency, whether voluntary or involuntary, is hardly the sole generator of ethical responsibility in a community or society. Vulnerability is also a stimulus to behavioral expectations. The usual formulation of an ethical principle which has its genesis in the relative vulnerability of one party in a relationship as compared with another, is of the order of: one does not (should not) take advantage of someone who is vulnerable in a relationship, or in a situation in which a relationship can be inferred—whether because of deficiencies in strength or intellectual capacity, or discretion, or experience, etc.

William [Willard] C. Richan's definition of client vulnerability in social work relationships can be generalized to apply to other relationships and thus be suited to its operation in other relationships. In his definition, vulnerability refers "to the susceptibility of people . . . to damage or exploitation stemming from incompetent or unethical behavior." Richan goes on to suggest that "This vulnerability may be something the client brings with him or may actually result from the kind of service being provided" (1961, p. 24).

---

[1] In spite of the restrictions frequently imposed on parents by the courts, parents have been accorded considerable latitude in relation to their children. Great discretion (Chaffin v. Chaffin, 1964) and a considerable amount of control (Termano v. Termano, 1965) have been adjudged essential for parents in the performance of their parental duty to provide for their children's support, discipline, and education. Principles of general ethics would nevertheless hold parents to a high standard of ethical responsibility.

Vulnerability may be brought by anyone to any relationship, whether the other person in the relationship is actually engaged in the provision of a service or not. It is the position, status, or influence of the other person that determines and affects the extent of one's vulnerability, and the potential for advantage and exploitation.

Kant provides an apt, if relatively innocuous, illustration of the vulnerability-advantage phenomenon in his case of the wayward tradesperson and the young or otherwise inexperienced customer. "It is always a matter of duty," Kant writes, "that a dealer should not overcharge an inexperienced purchaser" (Abbott, 1889, p. 31). He goes on to formulate a principle of ethical conduct which generalizes the expectation to all relationships between tradespersons and customers, so that the conduct is not contingent upon the vulnerability of the customer but is based rather on the expectation of consistency or the avoidance of discrimination. These are also principles of ethical practice, since they express preferences for one kind of behavior over another in particular relationships. The specific principle that Kant proposes is that "wherever there is much commerce the prudent tradesman does not overcharge, but keeps a fixed price for everyone, so that a child buys of him as well as any other. Men are thus honestly served."

Unfortunately for the purposes of this discussion, Kant proceeds to offer a practical basis for his principle when he explains that "this is not enough to make us believe that the tradesman has so acted from duty and from principles of honesty: his own advantage required it." The advantage to which Kant alludes is not specifically that over the overcharged and perhaps defenseless customer, but simply the self-interest of the tradesman in its own right. As Kant elaborates his point, "the action [of the tradesman] was done neither from duty nor from direct inclination, but merely with a selfish view."

Kant's emphasis on the practical considerations which he says inspires the tradesman's constraint, even when his opportunity for unfair advantage is an inviting one, prompts me to propose a requirement for administrative ethics. That requirement is that the behavior which is valued, and therefore appraised as ethical, is valued without regard to its prospectively practical consequences and advantages. Conduct in administrative practice which is appraised as "right" or "good" on the basis of espoused value is so appraised without regard to its practical outcome. This, at least, is what I propose to emphasize. And it applies to both the ends and the instrumentalities of administrative practice and behavior.

General ethics is relevant to administrative practice and behavior in that what is expected of people in general by way of ethical conduct is expected of all personnel associated with a social organization. This includes board members, professional staff, clerical staff, maintenance staff, and others. Because a social organization *is* a *social* organization and, to that extent, a part of its community and society, the expectations in ethical conduct which are normative in that community and society are applied to those associated with the organization and to the relationships and responsibilities in which and with which they are engaged.

Administration Is Everybody's Business in Social Organizations

Everyone who works for and in a social organization, or represents the organization, however informally, is assumed to share administrative responsibility in and for the organization. For some it is specifically assigned responsibility. For others it is delegated responsibility. For still others it is implied responsibility. And for a number of organizational personnel it is each of these at one time or another, and occasionally all of them. Some of the norms of a community or society which presumably guide the conduct of its members and which constitute criteria by which their conduct is evaluated with varying degrees of force and influence are specifically applicable to the administrative role and to administrative responsibility. They will therefore be specifically applicable to organizational personnel.

A social organization, moreover, is enough of a public entity, and sufficiently in the public eye, that actions in it and on its behalf are subject to public reaction, public concern, public scrutiny, and public intervention. If, for example, there is widespread indignation about corporate bribery (as there seems to be), there will be indignation among contributors to the coffers of a social organization if the personnel of that organization resort to bribes in order to outdistance other organizations in the competition for grants or allocations. The reaction to personnel of social organizations, in fact, is likely to be much more critical since the social norms in a country like the United States might allow for an occasional deviation in the interest of profit, an aspiration not associated with social organizations, and certainly not the professions which normally operate within them.

Whatever "isn't done" (in the sense of "ought not to be done") in the community or society at large will raise eyebrows if not ire and litigation when the personnel of social organizations do it.

Organizational Ethics

Organizational ethics defines the moral obligations of everyone in a social organization on the basis of the fact that the organization is in fact a social organization. Specific behavioral expectations are attributed to all organizational personnel, whether volunteer or paid, and whether professional or not, because of the purposes served by the organization, and because of the people affected by the organization as well as its purposes.

These expectations are distinguishable from the expectations associated with actual service relationships—the relationship between social worker and client, for example. This does not mean that the two sets of expectations never coincide, for they do at many points. A social worker incurs the obligation to safeguard the confidences of a client as does an administrator or a secretary in the social worker's employing organization. But the reasons are different. An entire set of "rules"—some more specific and explicit than others—governs the relationship between the social worker and the client. These "rules" have in fact been formalized by incorporation in codes of ethics adopted by professional social work organizations. As far as the relationship between a social organization as a whole and any of its clients is concerned, however, the ethical responsibility for safeguarding the client's confidences, which is ascribed to *any* representative of the organization by communal and social norms, results from the position of the organization in the community and society and its social function in both. The organization as an organization has an accounting to make for the actions of its personnel. Among other things, it is in this respect that the organization can be said to be guided and governed by principles of ethics.

In this connection, the legal concept of the technically constructed trust aptly describes the relationship between a social organization and its community. An organization can hardly have a relationship with a person, let alone a community, upon the basis of which ethical responsibility may be assumed or ascribed. However, such a relationship may be technically constructed to imply the incurring of such responsibility by anyone who runs, works for, or represents the organization. Moreover, that responsibility would affect not only persons and institutions with which the organization may already be dealing, but also persons and institutions with which the organization *might* deal. That responsibility would affect also those with whom the organization might have the obligation to deal; as well as others whom the organization might have the obligation to consider in its choices of action, procedures, and programs—prospective clients, for example.

These relationships upon which an organization's ethical responsibility is founded are "constructed" in that they are assumed to exist whether so defined or not. They therefore require behavioral constraints, or dictate affirmative expectations. As articulated in Troyak v. Enos:

> In Whitesell v. Striekler . . . the court said: ". . . in all cases where the relations in life are such that influence is acquired by one and confidence reposed by another, so as to give rise to opportunity for imposition or undue influence, such as arise between guardian and ward, parent and child, husband and wife, principal and agent, and the like, and where one of the parties, by reason of his surroundings, is unable to treat with the other upon terms of equality, courts of equity will carefully scrutinize the dealings with them and compel restoration in the absence of absolute fairness. . . ." [Bogert comments] "Obviously this constructive trust is not the product of the intent of the parties" (1953, p. 543).

Organizational ethics is of course not limited to the kind of fiduciary duty that was of primary concern in this case. Behavioral expectations based on the nature, relationships, and operations in and of a social organization range much more widely than that. They are nevertheless based on what the organization is and does, and why. How enforceable those expectations are is another matter, unless laws have been enacted to govern them. But they will figure in the awareness if not the consciences of those who manage the organization and those who work in and for it.

Whether or not the expectations operate as a constraint or influence on their conduct in their organizational capacity is also another matter. On the other hand, the expectations are likely to affect the reactions and the demands of others. In any case, they are relevant to organizational administration, since the relationships in and of the social organization are a critical component of organizational administration.

Organizational ethics is thus a formulation of behavioral expectations associated with the reason for an organization's existence, and the impact of the organization on human beings. An illustration is the expectation that a city department of social service will pay prompt and considerate attention to the income maintenance needs of persons who find themselves in dire financial straits. It is not only money that the department, through its personnel, is expected to provide but also—in the spirit of public assistance as a legislated right, and in the spirit of the kind of compassion that the Western tradition is supposed to be noted for—prompt attention to, and considerate treatment of applicants. On the one hand, the department is established to do a particular piece of work. The responsibility of its personnel to see to it that that work is done is both administrative and ethical. On the other hand, those who apply to the department to have that work done in their behalf are, to a great extent, disadvantaged because of their need to have it done. Personnel charged with doing the work are to some extent in a position of power in relation to the applicants. If they do not do the work, the applicants may be deprived of food, shelter, and other necessities of life.

Since the department exists to serve persons who are in financial need and physically and emotionally subject to the impact of that need, the responsibility of the department's personnel is both administrative and ethical. It is administrative in that administration, according to a traditional definition of the term, is the implementation of an organization's policies and functions. It is ethical in that certain modes of behavior in the implementation of those policies and functions are occupationally and socially valued, and others are disvalued.

Applicants kept waiting for hours outdoors on a cold, wintry day—as I have seen applicants to be at some welfare centers—while guards leisurely and tantalizingly wander about behind the closed doors, are subjected to a lapse in organizational ethics. Applicants kept aimlessly waiting in a cold and dismal waiting room while receptionists and clerks—the first to be encountered by the applicants—loquaciously relive their weekends and their love affairs while the applicants look helplessly and desolately on, are also subjected to a lapse in organizational ethics. The neglect by a clerk of required forms and other paraphernalia, so that financial assistance is inordinately delayed, and a measure of it perhaps lost forever although the hunger of the applicants persists, may also be regarded as a lapse in organizational ethics. Whatever the significance of these lapses for administrative responsibility, they also have ethical significance. Whatever other organizational and general norms are offended by these acts and omissions, they offend also what are readily formulated as principles of ethical conduct to which a social organization, and hence all of its personnel, may be assumed to be committed. All, moreover, emerge out of the position and function of the department of social service as a social organization.

A similar picture may be drawn of a hospital emergency room in which persons with alarming medical conditions, and with considerable anxiety about those conditions as well as other circumstances in their lives, are ignored for hours, their elemental physical needs like feeding and toileting being neglected and their very lives perhaps slipping away in the process. The function of providing health care is thus not performed, which may thus be regarded as an administrative failure. But this response, or the lack of it, to persons in physical and mental distress, may also be regarded as an ethical failure.

An illustration of a different order is the designing, by the leadership of a social organization, of arrangements and procedures which militate against access to service which the organization is established and chartered to provide. These arrangements might include locating the service at a place too distant, with transportation too expensive for clients for whom the service was ostensibly established; or setting hours so that poor working people, for whom the service is primarily intended, cannot resort to it without sacrificing more of their pitiful income than they can possibly afford. More will be said later about the bases as well as nature of the expectations implied in these cases and about the principles of ethical practice which may be formulated to reflect them.

Occupational Ethics

The third category of ethics under which the ethics of social work administration may be ordered—occupational ethics—begins to specify not so much the expectations attributed to social organizations as institutional entities, as is true of general ethics and organizational ethics, as the expectations attributed to administrators, at any level of administrative responsibility, specifically in their occupational capacity as administrators. In this context, administration may be regarded as an occupation in its own right with its own ethical specifications. It does appear from the rather extensive literature on management and administration in both industrial and social organizations that administration is guided by rather clearly enunciated principles of administrative practice. For administrators—that is, personnel employed and paid to perform administrative functions—these constitute occupational dicta, the "right" way to do the job in light of what is known about organizational processes and organization theory, and in light of what is known or hypothesized about what tends to work and not to work in the attainment of organizational goals and purposes. These principles presumably can be learned and taught so that individuals can become equipped to perform administrative functions and undertake administrative assignments at increasingly complex levels of administrative responsibility. These individuals presumably can also organize themselves to pursue common occupational interests and advance the state of administrative art.

When endeavors like administration attain such a stage their practitioners are in a position to identify and even to codify the values by which they choose collectively to be guided in the performance of administrative functions. There is enough commonality among them in what they do, regardless of where they do it, to make possible generalizations about their moral obligations as administrators and about preferences which they share regarding how they should treat and deal with others. It is not only what works that commands their attention, but also what they agree they owe to others by way of occupational duty. In these respects, the category of occupational ethics corresponds to ethics as it has been codified by a large number of professions, including social work.

The judgment of whether or not administration qua administration is a profession in its own right with its own code of ethics is not as vital to the purpose of this book as the development of an appreciation of what goes into the practice of administration in order to arrive at an understanding of the ethical responsibility applicable to that practice. What the category of occupational ethics suggests is that for a specific group of practitioners, for whom administration is a vocation for which they have some preparation, principles of ethical practice exist or may be formulated for which these practitioners may be held accountable in a manner in which others in social organizations may not—not at least in justice and equity.

On the other hand, there is nothing by way of general or organizational ethics for which others in social organizations may be held accountable that administrators in those organizations—which is to say practitioners who are occupationally identified as administrators and employed to perform administrative functions—are not. To put this more colloquially, administrators, for whom administration is a paid occupation, have all of the ethical responsibilities of the volunteer leadership of the social organizations by which they are employed, and then some. And for them, moreover, ethical responsibility is occupational responsibility and not only institutional responsibility.

Since I am addressing primarily the ethics of social work administration, another distinction merits emphasis. Social work administration is regarded here as the administration of social organizations, or organizations the function of which it is to provide social services of various kinds to those in need of them, and to afford social opportunities of various kinds for those who can make constructive use of them. Remembering this, one must also remember that although many administrators of social organizations are indeed social workers by identification and educational preparation, they need not be and many are not. Occupational ethics in the administration of social organizations is therefore not identical, and in some respects not even comparable with social work ethics.

This leads to an additive conception of the ethics of social work administration. Whatever the occupational identification of an administrator of a social organization, if other than administration but in addition to it, that administrator is accountable for the ethics of the occupation with which he or she is additionally identified. Either that, or the administrator must reconcile the ethics both of that occupation and of administration, to the extent that ethical responsibility can be ascribed or defined for both, or choose between them when they differ or are in conflict at any point. This applies, for example, when the occupation with which the administrator is identified is social work. The administrator is then bound by both social work and administrative ethics.

In a way, this is tantamount to double jeopardy, but that is one of the hazards of a dual identity. The administrator who belongs to a service occupation, whether social work or medicine or law or any other, and particularly one who expresses identification with it by formal membership and a commitment to its ethics, is subject to expectations for it and to the expectations ascribed to administrators.

Practitioners of various occupations are often employed to implement the service-related functions of social organizations. Community mental health centers, child guidance clinics, hospitals, sheltered workshops, settlement houses and community centers, family service agencies, and so on, employ social workers, psychiatrists, psychologists, vocational guidance counselors, and others. Each of these groups is guided by, or has ascribed to it, behavioral expectations adapted to the roles they perform in social organizations. Although these expectations focus on the relationship between practitioners and clients —and that not always sufficiently to suit consumers of their services who perceive them as being more concerned about one another than about their clients —although these expectations relate to clients, they generally also affect administrative relationships and responsibilities.

Such expectations, however, tend to be primarily designed to guide and govern the ethics of practitioners in the practice of their occupations rather than in administrative roles as such. Administrative ethics has to be largely extrapolated, or otherwise provided for. One way of providing for administrative ethics, of course, is to arrive at it independently. This would be a natural consequence of treating administration as a distinguishable occupation regardless of the collateral occupational identifications of administrators. But whether a practitioner of a service occupation is an administrator (additionally or exclusively) or not, that practitioner is properly (from a deontological point of view) expected to abide by the principles of ethical practice by which his or her service occupation is guided or governed. When the practitioner is an administrator, principles of ethical practice in administration also apply.

Since this is a book about administrative ethics, the principles of ethics that apply to the service component of an organization's functions may not appear to be germane. However, that dimension of administration which includes helping relationships between paid administrators and others makes such principles germane. An example of this dimension would be the relationship between a social agency's executive and the agency's board of directors, since it is the executive's assigned responsibility to help the board and its individual members to perform their organizational functions, and to relate to them in a way that makes the performance of those functions possible.

Although all paid personnel in a social organization share administrative responsibility at one level or another, not all share all administrative responsibilities of the same kinds at the same level. By the same token, neither do all share ethical responsibility of the same kind at the same level. But, in the administrative context as such (for they may be operating in other contexts as well), all carry ethical responsibility of some kind at some level. That responsibility stems from the kind of administrative responsibility that they share.

All paid administrators—personnel for whom administration is assigned occupational responsibility and for whom specifiable preparation is prescribed and required—carry ethical responsibility of a nature specifiable in relation to those with whom they deal and what they are accountable for as a result. Whereas the ethical responsibility of volunteers in a social organization—whether policy-makers or program participants—is a function of the relationship between the social organization and its community and society, the ethical responsibility of administrative staff is a function of the job they are vocationally assigned to do.

The ethical responsibility of program and policy-making volunteers in a social organization is a function of voluntarily assumed positions in the organization. The ethical responsibility of administrative staff is a function of their status as organization employees and as practitioners with a specific occupational identity. Although the ethical responsibility of administrative staff is apt to be more inclusive than that of volunteers, the ethical responsibility of volunteers—the responsibility which may be attributed to them because of their roles in the social organization—is not, by virtue of their status at any rate, in any degree dispensable.

For those for whom administration is an occupational responsibility in a social organization, ethics can be codified to the extent that it can be codified for any occupation that can be functionally differentiated from other occupations. For those for whom administrative responsibility is voluntarily assumed in the public or in a social interest, principles of ethics may be proposed—as I shall be attempting to do—as a matter of social responsibility, social control, and social constraint.

For administrative staff, ethical responsibility is part of "the job" of administration. For volunteers, ethical responsibility is part of the way of social life in a community or society, and in a social organization, given the purposes that the social organization serves in that community or society and the role it plays there.

One reason for the emphasis on these distinctions is that what may be attributed to volunteers in an organization by way of the niceties of ethical conduct because of the positions of trust they hold in behalf of their community, must be regarded as ethical imperatives for administrative staff at all levels of administrative responsibility. What is a generous gesture on the part of volunteers, which nevertheless generates ethical encumbrances (I leave aside here the more exploitative motivations which prompt volunteers to offer their wisdom, their resources, and their services), is a way of working life for the administrative staff of social organizations.

Whatever the variations among social organizations with respect to size, scope, purpose, sponsorship, auspices, sources of support, etc., there is a common enough base of administrative operation and practice to make possible and valid common guides to ethical conduct on the part of administrators in them, although there may be some basis for some differentiation among them, less as far as basic principles of ethical practice are concerned than particular applications of those principles.

Differentials in Ethical Responsibility

Differentiation may be necessary with respect to the principles which apply to administrators in social organizations, and the intensity with which they apply, as a result of their position in the administrative hierarchy of the organization. One reason for this is that their authority varies on that basis, as do the relationships which their responsibility makes possible and necessary. Relative power is a critical variable in the process of differentiation. Again, it is not necessarily the principles of ethical practice which change so much as their operation and application. The importance of an administrator's ethics is obviously affected by the administrator's opportunities to be unethical, and with whom.

In short, a different order of administrative ethics would appear to be required not only as between volunteers and paid administrators, but also as between chief executives and sub-executives; and as between administrators and other organizational personnel. Similarly, differentiation would appear to be required as between professional personnel and nonprofessional personnel.

Further differentiation may be necessary with respect to ethical responsibility in relation to internal organizational practice and external organizational practice—that is, behavior expected, on ethical grounds, in the relationships among organizational personnel, and that in the relationships of organizational personnel to others outside of the organization. Often these do not coincide, and sometimes they clash irreconcilably. As with ethics in general, and notably occupational ethics, a modicum of discretion is required and expected and must be scrupulously exercised, just as it must when two or more ethical responsibilities conflict enough so that both cannot be accommodated. This, too, merits further attention and will receive it.

Finally, before I venture into some of the substantive aspects of the ethics of social work administration, I should like to offer an additional distinction—that between management and administration—since I shall be focusing on the latter and not the former. These concepts are often used interchangeably, but they do warrant differentiation, at least for the present purpose. I would like to limit the concept of management to the operational processes involved in running an organization. The primary connotation in this conception is the concern and contention of practitioners with "things."[2] These include computers, budgets, accounts, equipment, recorded policies and plans, money, plant, etc. Administration, on the other hand, will be used here to signify organizational and occupational relationships to persons and organizations engaged in, or affected by, all of the processes and procedures of a social organization, including the "things" that they deal with in order to get the organization's work done, the resources required to get that work done, and the accountings that are called for in relation to both. My intention in making these distinctions is to accentuate that component of the organizational enterprise—particularly that in social organizations—to which ethics is most, and perhaps peculiarly, relevant.

What I propose to do now is to consider the ethics prescriptively attributable to all personnel in social organizations—volunteer or paid, professional or nonprofessional. I shall also consider the premises for such attribution. The range of considerations should include the nature of the ethical responsibility attributable to all personnel as it may be derived from the nature and purposes of social organizations, and that responsibility as it may be derived from the nature of the functions, positions, and status of those personnel in the organi-

---

[2]Although this conception of management is not derived from Martin Heidegger, his analysis of "thing" and "thingness" appears to be intriguingly pertinent to it. One of his answers to his question, "What is a thing?" is "A thing is the existing (*vorhanden*) bearer of many existing (*vorhanden*) yet changeable *properties*" (emphasis added; 1967, p. 34). In alluding to the results of his inquiry into the question, he goes on to refer to the "frame of the thing, time-space, and the thing's way of encountering, the 'this,' and then the structure of the thing itself as being the bearer of properties, entirely general and empty" (p. 53). Apropos of the development of modern science, he says, "the thing is material, a point of mass in motion in the pure space-time order, or an appropriate combination of such points. . . . *The animate is also here.* Even where one permits the animate its own character, it is conceived as an *additional* structure built upon the inanimate" (emphases added, which I also take to signify a distinction from things; p. 51).

zations. If this much can be successfully done, it may then be useful to consider approaches to implementation of such ethics as may be prescribed for social work administration, particularly for organization executives, and for education in relation to it.

REFERENCES

Abbott, Thomas Kingsmill, Trans. *Kant's Critique of Practical Reason And Other Works on The Theory of Ethics* (Fourth ed. rev.; London: Longmans, Green, 1889).

Chaffin v. Chaffin, 397 P. 2nd 771 (1964).

Heidegger, Martin. *What Is A Thing?* Trans. W. W. Barton, Jr. and Vera Deutsch, with an analysis by Eugene T. Gendlin (Chicago: Henry Regnery, 1967).

Richan, William C. "A Theoretical Scheme for Determining Roles of Professional and Nonprofessional Personnel," *Social Work*, 6 (1961), 22-28.

Termano v. Termano, 205 N.E. 2nd 586, 1 Ohio App. 2nd 504 (1965).

Troyak v. Enos, 204 F. 2nd 536 (1953).

III. THE ETHICS OF SOCIAL ORGANIZATIONS

Amitai Etzioni begins his little gem of a book, *Modern Organizations,* with a statement which serves especially well as a starting point for this chapter:

> Our society is an organizational society. We are born in organizations, educated by organizations, and most of us spend much of our lives working for organizations. We spend much of our leisure time paying, playing, and praying in organizations. Most of us will die in an organization, and when the time comes for burial, the largest organization of all—the state—must grant official permission (1964, p. 1).

Knowledge and Values in Relation to Organizations and Administration

There are many kinds of organizations, of course, but this statement reflects the extent to which social organizations figure in our lives, affect our lives, and influence the directions which our lives take. There is much that is known about social organizations and about organizations in general, profit-making and antisocial organizations (for example, the Ku Klux Klan and street gangs) included. There is also much that can and needs to be known about organizations if ethics in them and of them is to be understood and provided for.

But knowledge about organizations, as about administration, is only a basis for understanding the ethics of social work administration and of administration in general—only the context within which ethics and the need for it can be understood and principles of ethical behavior can be formulated. As Herbert Simon and his colleagues once put it:

> Knowledge of administration, like all knowledge, is amoral. It becomes "good" or "bad" only in terms of the value assumptions added to it by the person who uses it—in terms of his attitudes towards goals and methods. Knowledge gives man power—but power to do either good or evil. . . . Knowledge of administration is amoral in an even deeper sense, for it is knowledge of how to manipulate other human beings—how to get them to do the things you want done. The study of administration discloses techniques for influencing human behavior (Simon, Smithburg, and Thompson, 1958, p. 22).

More affirmatively, knowledge of and about organizations as well as administration can be used as a basis for proposing guides to ethical conduct in social organizations. Since organizations are constructed as they are, and operate as they do, and since administrators and other organization personnel have a lot to do with what organizations do and how they do it, what is known about both can be converted into behavioral aspirations. What is valued about what organizations and their personnel do can be expressed as expectations and desiderata regarding what they *should* do. Moreover, under an effective system of informal as well as formal social control,[1] they can be judged and even disciplined if they do not do it. Viewed more positively, however, the knowledge which has been and can be accumulated about organizations and administration may be employed to reach for the stars, as it were—to reach for idealizations of organizational and administrative conduct which are not manifest and which nobody expects to be realized at a particular time or place but which are nevertheless valued, encouraged, and the object of social recognition and reward. "The progress of knowledge," Pierre Du Noüy has written, "should be encouraged to the extent that it can serve action, or the moral elevation of man, and not as a mere means of acquiring knowledge" (1966, p. 184). Distinguishing scientific law and social law, Du Noüy emphasizes the fact that, unlike scientific law, "the social law is an arbitrary rule established a priori and possesses an absolute authority based on the interest of the community and perhaps also on a kind of innate idea which is very difficult to define but is nevertheless powerful; namely justice" (p. 189).[2]

The values of and for a social organization, and the behaviors which are valued for its personnel in relation to one another and to others—which is to say their ethics—are in a sense arbitrary. They are *chosen* by the organization

---

[1] E. A. Ross's early analysis of social control is much too inclusive in its scope to be resorted to here. Some of his observations are nevertheless quite applicable, among them the following: "There are three bodies of feeling and opinion that work together in shaping social control; namely, that of those who wish to follow a certain line of conduct, that of those who are injured by such conduct, and that of the rest of the community. The second and third *impose* control, the first *limits* it" (1969, p. 62). "A control that we have any right to call *social* has behind it practically the whole weight of society. But still this control often wells up and spreads out from certain centres which we might term *the radiant points of social control*" (p. 77). Such instruments of social control as public opinion, suggestion, personal ideal, social religion, art, and social valuation draw their strength from the primal moral feelings. They take their strength from sentiment rather than utility. They control men in many things which have little to do with the welfare of society regarded as a corporation. They are aimed to realize not merely a social order, but what might be termed a *moral* order. These we may call ethical" (p. 411).

[2] In this connection, it is interesting to note the themes which Abraham Kaplan identifies as recurring elements in the various world philosophies, and which he explains to be but a few useful "guides to the understanding of what most of these philosophies are getting at" (1961, p. 7). The themes he identifies are rationality; activism ("understanding is not sufficient unto itself but serves as a guide to action. . . . Knowledge [provides] us . . . with a map by which to find our way"—p. 8); humanism ("the centrality of man in the philosophy itself, if not in the world philosophised about"—p. 9); and values ("the basis on which values can be grounded"—p. 9). It is obvious, that what we are about here is more philosophy than science; more values than facts. Science and facts—knowledge—are the grounding for the values to be suggested however forcefully—suggested, not proven—in relation to administrative conduct.

and its personnel or by others who, individually or institutionally, may or may not be in agreement about them. The values are chosen as preferable to other values and valued behaviors. But they may be validated by an analysis of organizational circumstances and operations and their potential consequences— that is, by knowledge about the organization and the relationships and situations to which the organization's purpose and functions give rise.

The Ethics of Social Organizations

The question which organizational ethics primarily addresses is: under the circumstances and in the situations which emerge in a social organization as a consequence of its freedom and responsibility to perform specific functions in a community and society, what may reasonably be expected or required of its personnel by way of ethical conduct in relation to others served or affected by what is done in and on behalf of the organization, and what is not done as well? Also of concern is what is or is not done in relation to others with a personal or institutional stake in both. Such behavioral expectations or requirements must, of course, "make sense" in light of the purpose and functions of the social organization, and in light of the interest of others affected by both, including the community and the society.

The "others" to whom a social organization owes ethical responsibility include clients, organization staff, volunteers, contributors to the organization's support, prospective clienteles for whom the organization's services and programs may become revelant if they are not already, interorganizational structures of which the organization is a constituent part or to which it owes some kind of accounting, etc. The others are not only those with whom the organization, through its personnel, deals, but also those with whom the organization *might* deal, or *ought* to deal, given its purpose and its functions as well as its circumstances.

As I have already suggested, organizations as organizations do not *do anything,* or *relate* to *anybody.* It is their personnel at any and all levels, volunteer or paid, who do both. And if it can be said that organizations owe ethical responsibility—and that can indeed be said—it is through their personnel that this responsibility is expressed and implemented. The focus of the present discussion, however, is the ethical responsibility of the social organization as a corporate entity. The immediate question to be explored, therefore, is: what is it that the social organization owes by way of ethical responsibility, and to whom, in view of its purpose and functions and the sanction and support of the community and society for both? What is there about what social organizations are and do, and what they are relied upon by others to be and to do, that implies ethical responsibility on the part of everyone and anyone associated with them? And, what are the nature and implications of that responsibility?

The initial premise for the determination of the kind of ethical responsibility that may justifiably be attributed to social organizations as such, is suggested by Etzioni when he says that, "Organizations are social units (or human groupings) deliberately constructed and reconstructed to seek specific goals" (1964, p. 3), and particularly when he adds that "organizations are much more in control of their nature and destiny than any other social grouping."

The goals of a social organization, as Etzioni suggests, provide guidelines for the activities in and of the organization. But they "also constitute a source of legitimacy which justifies the activities of an organization and, indeed, its very existence" (p. 5). Herein lies the tale of organizational ethics, for that which is socially legitimated, including the creation, existence, and operation of a social organization, requires a social accounting. You cannot, in social control terms, have one without the other.

A social organization cannot be permitted, by the community and society, to do anything it pleases as an organization, not after the organization has been permitted by the community and society to exist and to function in specified and agreed upon ways, an act which itself requires particular care in the first place. Whether the permission is given via charter or informal sanction—by simply letting the organization happen, for example—the social organization is committed to the terms of that permission. Though these terms are seldom narrowly defined, or defined in particularistic detail, the purposes and functions to which they apply are generally quite clear. They do not specify how the organization's work is to be done, but they do indicate *what* that work is.

The sanction accorded to a social organization, whether formal or informal, may depend on what the organization seeks to do and why. Some organizations acquire what amounts to residual sanction. The purposes of the Ku Klux Klan, for example, are not generally approved and yet that organization is permitted to function although subject to such legal constraints as all others are. However, what is sanctioned—and there are many who would not begrudge the organization that much—is not so much its stated purposes, which do run counter to democratic norms because of the bigotry implicit in them, as the freedom of expression for its members, which also happens to be valued in the United States. Thus, what is socially sanctioned is not what the Ku Klux Klan chooses to do but its legal right to do it. Beyond that, the fate of the organization will rest either on the operation of the law, or on the responses of the community. If its members break the law by violence, vandalism, or the deprivation of the constitutional rights of others, they and the organization will have to answer for that. If they offend the ethical norms of enough of the community's constituents, the organization may lose members and financial support. But for the latter to occur, ethical norms have to exist, and they have to be subscribed to with sufficient scope and intensity to have an appreciable effect on either the behavior of the organization, or the responses of others.

A social organization which is accorded community and societal sanction for the purposes and functions it has decided to address, incurs the moral obligation to hew closely to those purposes and functions—until, at least, it earns the sanction for new or different ones. This is ethical responsibility. It is analogous to the promise one individual makes to another on which the latter relies, for what one promises, one has the ethical responsibility to do. If reasons emerge for not doing it, then the failure to do it must be justified on grounds comprehensible to others. But it must be regarded as a failure in ethical terms. What one is implying in failing to fulfill a promise is that, despite the acknowledged obligation to fulfill it, practical or philosophical considerations are regarded as justifying the failure to do so. But it would take some kind of adjudication or evaluation to determine whether those considerations were sufficiently compelling to justify or excuse the failure.

Ethics as a Function of Organizational Purpose

A social organization is expected to do what it has been established to do because that is what it has led the community and society to expect of it. It is unethical not to do it.

This major premise leads ineluctably to a chain of additional premises, some not so minor depending upon the intensity with which certain values are espoused and the circumstances in which they figure. The neglect of starving children by a child welfare agency charged by charter or consensus to feed them, for example, will no doubt be responded to by a community with greater indignation than the serving of junk food for lunch in a day care center. It is a principle of organizational ethics, based on general and communal expectations if not also on defined institutional function, that the organization address the purposes and implement the functions for which it has avowedly been created.

This is certainly true of social organizations, but it is also true of industrial and other profit-making organizations. General Motors may conglomerate itself *ad nauseum,* but as long as it remains General Motors it is expected to manufacture automobiles. True, the ultimate objective for this activity is to make a profit, but the road to profit is the production and sale of automobiles. The general public would not take kindly to the company's diversifying during a period of drooping sales to the point of sacrificing automobile production altogether and reconverting its real property into tobacco farms and its plants into cigarette factories—not at least without a satisfactory reason and the avowal of a new purpose which can then independently meet the test of community and social sanction.

The Merits of Organizational Purposes

For a social organization which veers off into a purpose other than the one which it has explicitly or implicitly promised, the offense to organizational ethics is all the greater to the extent that the purpose abandoned or neglected represents a pressing social need and the purpose assumed a relative luxury. In short, organizational ethics is offended by both the neglect of a purpose to which the organization has committed itself—and a purpose presumably sanctioned by the community as meriting attention—and the assumption of a purpose for which there is little or no perceived social need or justification. An equally serious· problem in organizational ethics would be introduced if the purpose continued to be honored but, instead of being honored in relation to a population in need for whom the purpose was originally intended, the purpose were redirected to benefit a population perceived to be less in need of its implementation or not in need of its implementation at all.

Consider as an example a community center which was originally established in a slum area to provide for the recreational and developmental needs of poor immigrant families and impoverished members of ethnic minority groups. To get more support, and to appeal to a more affluent constituency, the center relocates in a distant suburb, and constructs a luxurious health club replete with saunas and massage tables. The center, of course, also increases its membership and program fees. It does offer scholarships but they are not likely to be helpful to those who need the scholarships but cannot make it to the new neighborhood.

The center is still providing recreational and developmental services, just as it originally promised, although with slight variations—but for whom? The "for whom?" is as relevant a question of organizational ethics for a social organization as the "what" of its purpose.

This suggests an additional issue in organizational ethics, a perhaps more controversial one in view of the valuation of autonomy—including organizational autonomy—in western society and particularly in the United States. This issue has to do with the very choice of organization purpose and function in the first place.

It would seem to be self-evident that—aside from considerations of law, and ethical considerations *are* aside from law though sometimes governed by law— it would seem to be self-evident that social organizations would not be encouraged if they sought sanction for a destructive purpose. Such a purpose, in fact, would be regarded as unethical in the context of what, as a social organization, it would be regarded as owing by way of duty to its community and society.

Even profit-making organizations are constrained when what they propose or purport to do is manifestly harmful to persons or to a community. The manufacture and advertising of cigarettes were for a long time unrestricted until cigarette smoking was found in some research to be carcinogenic. Community values were evidently not influential enough to wipe out the powerful cigarette industry, but sufficiently influential to effect the requirement of an inscribed warning on each package of cigarettes regarding their potential hazard for smokers. The ambiguity of the underlying values affecting the manufacture and sale of cigarettes makes it impossible to judge either process to be unethical.

On the other hand, there is a kind of ethical nod implicit in the required warning. It may not be unethical to make and sell cigarettes, given the present state of values and behavioral expectations derived from them, but it might be unethical not to offer the caution about them—even if the law did not require as much.

Other activities less normative in the society might not be tolerated even that much, and might be subjected to a less equivocal characterization as unethical. Antisocial purposes would be so characterized since social organizations are expected to perform functions which serve the purposes of society, not militate against them. Real estate block-busting to restrict the housing opportunities of minority group members—even if scrupulously attentive to legal mandate— would be regarded as unethical in the context of organizational ethics since housing organizations share the duty of fairness to all who have need of housing, and the duty not to discriminate against persons because of their religion or skin color.[3] Social organizations would certainly be expected to be responsive to these duties precisely because they are social organizations, the presumption being that they serve and do not disserve social purposes.

There are more subtle demands that may be imposed on social organizations as dicta of organizational ethics, also on the basis of the presumption that social organizations are expected—since they have the ethical responsibility as social organizations—to serve social purposes, and certainly not to obstruct them.[4]

Social organizations, for one thing, are not free, as a matter of ethics, to choose any social purpose they please, even if they do not intend to draw on the resources of their community to support the purpose they prefer. This principle of organizational ethics which I am proposing applies even when the purpose preferred is also social in that it provides for a service or program which is quite constructive. The purpose may even be designed for a clientele which has need of that service or program, or can make productive use of it.

The fundamental consideration regarding the selection of a purpose for a social organization, or for creating or modifying a social organization in order to fulfill that purpose, is that the purpose selected be worthy of choice from the point of view of existing social and human need, and that it merit priority in relation to other necessary purposes if all cannot be concurrently served.

The issue to be contended with in implementing the organization's ethical

---

[3]The reader is reminded that such dicta are entirely prescriptive and not presumed to be empirically founded or a realistic account of current practice. On the other hand, there is considerable basis for relying on the values upon which prescriptive ethical dicta may be founded.

[4]Whatever may be expected of any actor by way of ethical duty, or any other kind of responsibility the fulfillment of which constitutes ethical duty—whatever, that is, represents affirmative expectations—the minimal expectation which may be codified as a principle of ethical conduct is that the actor will do nothing to subvert or obstruct the performance of that duty. A president charged with upholding the United States Constitution, for example, is ethically supercharged not to violate it or obstruct the enforcement of its provisions. Social organizations and individuals in them are similarly constrained on the basis of their defined responsibilities.

responsibility to its community and society is whether the choice of a social purpose is a valid one in its own right and in relation to alternatives. Among valid social purposes would be included protective services for children deprived of parental care or in physical danger because of the kind of care available to them; income maintenance for families in financial distress; health care for elderly persons with catastrophic and chronic illnesses; etc. Such purposes must be served if the well-being of a society and the people who compose it is to be provided for. But also of ethical concern is the choice of a social purpose that does not have the effect of tapping a community's resources, energy, attention, and so on, which are required for a more urgent purpose. This is of course reminiscent of the economic concept of opportunity cost: what is used for one purpose is not available for another.

These issues are hardly simple. Who is to judge whether a swimming pool for poor neighborhood children is less important or of less value than a program of foster care? Or whether discussion groups for lonely elderly persons are less important or of less value than a nursing home for incapacitated elderly persons? Or whether a social action organization for unemployed Hispanic persons is less important or of less value than a community theater group? On the other hand, judgments are required, especially when choices of purposes to be served must be made and not all choices can be realistically accommodated. Naturally, it would be better if the value of all such organizational purposes could be acknowledged and if, rather than ordering such purposes hierarchically, resources could be unearthed and developed to make possible the realization of all the purposes for which any real need can be certified to exist and to merit prompt attention. There is room in our society for services and programs with preventive, developmental, inspirational, esthetic, and other similarly affirmative purposes, and not only crisis-oriented, problem-related, clinical, rehabilitative, and corrective purposes.

The Purposes of Business and Industrial Organizations

The purposes and functions of business and industrial organizations are subject to the effects of competition and consumer response, however implausible and invalid such effects may sometimes be. Whether the purposes and functions of such organizations will be honored in a community or society, and whether the organizations which serve them will be maintained on a profitable basis, will be influenced by the capacity of the organizations to survive and flourish in the face of competition, and to affect the readiness, willingness, and ability of consumers to patronize them and compensate them.

The initiation, promotion, and endurance of business and industrial purposes and functions—including services as well as the manufacture of consumer products—will be sufficiently determined in most circumstances by consumer response, which can of course be influenced and precipitated by a sturdy advertising campaign and perhaps other methods for which business ethics is supposed to be a guide and constraint. Public policy is also an occasional constraint. More commonly, however, people vote with their feet and their funds, as it were, and some purposes and functions are elected and others are not. And in the wings, sometimes, hovers a Ralph Nader or a John Gardner to insure the consideration of values that consumers might not provide for on their own initiative.

Consumer response is often also a variable affecting the determination of whether the purposes and functions of social organizations can be initiated, promoted, and maintained; nor is the intrinsic merit of either purposes or functions invariably the critical consideration determining their fate.

Government and taxes may play a decisive role in the process through the establishment and support of public agencies for the implementation of necessary purposes and functions, but even then their intrinsic merit, or even their relative merit in comparison with other possible choices, is not always the most influential determinant. Politics and the legislative process have a way of circumventing the natural ebb and flow of values, and certainly the application of rationality to the process of weighing values against one another. As with business and industry, no less than commercial entertainment and artistic ventures, advertising, prestige, and publicity sometimes make the difference for the purposes and functions of social organizations as well.

But these are only the determinants of whether or not the purposes and functions of social organizations will or will not "take." The ethical issue for social organizations is whether or not they should undertake particular purposes and functions in the first place in the light of existing needs and the capacity of the community and society to provide for them. It is on these grounds, and on the basis of the responsibility of social organizations to their community and society, that social organizations incur their moral obligations.

Finding, Defining, and Implementing Social Purposes

Social organizations which seek to serve a social purpose, and seek community and societal support and sanction in relation to that purpose, are inevitably accountable for the accurate enunciation and clarification of that purpose, and for the demonstration of the need for it and of their capacity to meet that need. This is necessary for both the validation of its selection and the assurance to the community and society that they can manage the purpose both satisfactorily and in consonance with conceded community and societal values. It is also a matter of internal interest to the organizations as well as external interest to others that the organizations fulfill their purpose as proficiently and economically as possible, through the optimal employment of their human and material resources. A fundraising organization which raises funds for distribution to social organizations, for example, is expected to limit the amount of money it expends in order to raise those funds. Its ethics is open to question if it spends a disproportionate amount of money for this purpose, and if it raises funds in communally or societally disvalued ways. As is true of ethics in general, and certainly the ethics of social work administration, it is not only what is done but how it is done that counts for the purposes of organizational ethics.

A social organization presumably retains jurisdiction over its own policies, and presumably enjoys autonomy regarding its choice of purpose as well as its approach to the implementation of that purpose. Nevertheless, it has the ethical responsibility to consider the needs and preferences of its community and society, or at least that segment of both to which its purpose and functions may be relevant, or which they may affect, if only inadvertently. The organization also has the ethical responsibility to so organize itself that it can fulfill its assumed mission when that mission is in fact undertaken, and to demonstrate that it is in fact being fulfilled as promised. These are moral as well as practical obligations.

Organizational Autonomy Versus Organizational Responsibility

The prior question nevertheless remains—the autonomy of the social organization notwithstanding—and that relates to the very choice of what the organization does and why. By this I do not mean the personal motivations of the individuals who establish the organization—an issue in the ethics of social work administration which does deserve some attention. I mean, rather, the reasons for establishing the organization and undertaking the purposes to be served by it, as those reasons would be of concern to a community and society and affect both.

The moral obligation of social organizations to insure for all persons access to necessary services and programs corresponds to John Rawls' theory of justice which provides for the equalization of social opportunities for all while providing for the special needs of deprived and disadvantaged persons and groups (1971). This obligation applies in relation to all, however powerless they may be, however oppressed they may be, however impoverished they may be, if not because of those very circumstances. It applies in relation to those who are obscured in the crevices of urban life; or so removed from some of the more visible centers of urban life that they are easily overlooked altogether; or studiously ignored as inconsequential. It applies in relation to those who, in their filth and in their diseases, are unpalatable to decision-makers; who, in their values, are suspect to decision-makers. This moral obligation to consider such persons and weigh their needs, even when they cannot represent those needs themselves, is an awesome social responsibility, an intimidating ethical responsibility. Implicit in such responsibility, as it may be ascribed to social organizations, is a component of what Jane Addams so long ago described as social ethics:

All about us are men and women who have become unhappy in regard to their attitude toward the social order itself. . . . These men and women have caught a moral challenge raised by the exigencies of contemporaneous life . . . all are increasingly anxious concerning their actual relations to the basic organization of society. The test which they would apply to their conduct is a social test. They fail to be content with the fulfillment of their family and personal obligations, and find themselves striving to respond to a new demand involving a *social* obligation; they have become conscious of another requirement, and the contribution they would make is toward a *code of social ethics* (1964, pp. 3-4; emphasis supplied).[5]

The end-in-view of social ethics, or the kind of social obligation which may be attributed to social organizations, is social justice, which, David Miller has written, "concerns the distribution of benefits and burdens throughout a society, as it results from the major social institutions" (1976, p. 22). Miller includes under the rubric of social justice "the allocation of housing, medicine, welfare benefits, etc." Having included punishments within the scope of legal justice, Miller suggests that "'burdens' should be read to mean 'disadvantages other than punishments'—i.e., such things as unpleasant or onerous work, bad housing conditions, etc." (p. 22).

Miller does exclude power from the benefits subsumed under social justice. However, he goes on to admit that:

This is not to say of course that the distribution of power is irrelevant to social justice since the allocation of other benefits may in practice depend upon the shape of the power structure, but all this means is that the distribution of power is *causally* rather than *conceptually* relevant to social justice (p. 22).

Miller elaborates "benefits" to include "intangible benefits such as prestige and self-respect," and although, for his purposes, he considers "mainly material goods, especially wealth, which most people would consider the most important concern of social justice," these inclusions on Miller's part are significant, since they show that social organizations address intangible as well as tangible benefits. Social ethics, and therefore organizational responsibility, would require of social organizations well-considered and equitable choices of purpose as well as functions, particularly since the capacity to choose and sustain both represents an awesome source of power. Organizational ethics, on the other hand, makes imperative the considerate and judicious use of that power. Power

---

[5]Social ethics is equivalent to social responsibility in general and not to be confused with behavioral expectations or moral obligations associated with specific organizational and occupational responsibility and relationships to others.

inheres as well in the authorization to implement chosen purposes and functions, for organizations so sanctioned are strategically located to determine who does and who does not benefit from those purposes and functions, and under what conditions.

When subject to community planning and priorities, or to public and social policy, the social organization is not ethically at liberty to become an organization, let alone unilaterally to choose its own purposes and functions, or its own approach to their implementation. The organization may be ethically subject to policy and planning priorities even when it intends to rely on its own resources and not to resort to public or community funds.

The less independent a social organization is, the more subject to evaluation by others is its choice of mission. But, independent or not, the social organization as a social organization has the ethical responsibility to weigh its choice in relation to other possible choices affecting human need, not only as the organization sees it but also as the community and the society see it. For the organization, as well as the community and society, it boils down to a question of values: what is preferred to what and for whom? For justice and equity to be done, the negotiation of differences with respect to such values should be unbiased and systematic—behind the kind of veil of ignorance which John Rawls recommended, meaning of course not without data—quite to the contrary—but without bias and vested interest:

> The idea of the original position is to set up a fair procedure so that any principles agreed to will be just. The aim is to use the notion of pure procedural justice as a basis of theory. Somehow we must nullify the effects of specific contingencies which put men at odds and tempt them to exploit social and natural circumstances to their own advantage. Now in order to do this I assume that the parties are situated behind a veil of ignorance. They do not know how the various alternatives will affect their own particular case and they are obliged to evaluate principles solely on the basis of general considerations (1971, pp. 136-137).

Criteria to guide that process of negotiation and analysis would include who is in need of what that represents the greatest relative risk to life, health, interpersonal relationships, educational and employment opportunities, and so on. For the social organization such criteria are based on those to whom the organization has moral obligations.

A social organization in search of broad-scaled support—that is, not from a particular ethnic, cultural, or common-interest group—is certainly obliged to be guided in its choice of mission by the full range of existing social and human needs. It is obliged to select that need which is most pervasive and most inclusive in the scope of its effect; and that need which is either most neglected or most urgent; as well as that need which affects the most defenseless persons and groups, and those most exposed to danger and deprivation. The number of persons affected must of course also be considered, although minority groups, like disabled and chronically ill persons, must not be neglected because of their relatively limited numbers. Persons with comparatively less access to services and programs require particular consideration, whether their limitations are a consequence of insufficient funds or insufficient mobility.

A social organization content to confine itself to support from a homogeneous but limited group would appear to be ethically freer to pinpoint its purposes and functions to benefit that group. Ethnic, religious, and other groups are supposed to be accorded the right as well as privilege to provide for the needs of their own members. It was once an expectation in fact. Peter Stuyvesant set that as a condition for the admission of Jews to New York when it was under Dutch rule, and it remains a requirement for other immigrants. A social organization which exercises such an option is nevertheless ethically obliged to take into account the social welfare requirements of the community and the society as a whole, and to share responsibility along with other social organizations for meeting those requirements, not necessarily at the expense of legitimate in-group needs but, on the other hand, not to meet those needs at the expense of other more urgent ones.

The ethical responsibility of a social organization to address general as well as specific needs, or to provide for specific needs but to make programs for them more generally accessible and not limited to the group for whom they might have been originally designed, amounts to a moral pressure. The responsibility to improve effectiveness of the social welfare structure of a community and society in general is shared by other social organizations. The responsibility extends far enough to include the abandonment of sanctioned missions, and the modification of missions, as social needs and conditions change to require a reordering of social priorities. None of this means that what has been described actually happens—only that the ethical responsibility is incurred to make it happen.

When the choice of an organization's purpose and function is not at issue, either through organizational inertia or persevering conviction, a change in approach may be obligatory because the organization's methods and procedures do not work well, or do work but at inordinate cost in human and material resources, or in personal, organizational, social, and other consequences. It is then an ethical responsibility for the organization, as an organization, to reexamine not only what it aims to do but also how it is being done. The behaviorally expressed inclination of a social organization to maintain and preserve itself as it is—a rather common inclination—would have to be regarded as unethical.

An incident which occurred some years ago is dramatically illustrative of the ethical as well as policy implications and consequences of organizational choice regarding purpose and function. On the basis of work done by the Policy

Committee on Services to Groups of the Metropolitan Detroit United Community Services, Robert Vinter identified several "central issues" which, though represented as "findings" (i.e., facts), were really charged with preferential judgments:

1. We challenge the belief that group work and recreation (or, as it is more recently termed, "group services") is a unitary field.
2. The character of existing group services has not been adequately delineated nor rationally and equitably ordered for planning purposes.
3. The structure of administration and coordination of these services reflect an earlier era in community development and merit substantial modification.
4. The relation of the group services to other health and welfare services is poorly articulated, both at the level of service usage by clientele and at the level of inter-agency coordination (1961, p. 49).

Vinter then alluded to "some of the more pressing policy issues implicit in these service patterns," which he associated with a "major problem that has plagued policy formation and decisions about the allocation of scarce resources in the socialization area" (p. 57).

Here is the presentation of "evidence" (which is the description used in the title of Vinter's account) and the framing of policy issues, both of which are offered as premises for the resolution of the issues and for the formulation of policy by organization decision-makers. Whether an organization will take them seriously will depend on the autonomy it actually enjoys and its moral stake in the general community or social plan. Interorganizational and community pressure may do the job, but so may the collective conscience within the organization itself. The organization may not "listen," but it is ethically obliged to do so, and to consider and act upon what it hears. Once doubt has been cast upon what an organization has chosen to do and why the organization continues to do it in the way the organization has been doing it, the organization incurs the ethical responsibility to take an additional look at both, first because it may no longer be valid—which is to say, valued—and secondly because something else may have become more valid or more necessary.

Patti and Resnick reinforce this ethical judgment in their analysis of the provocations to organizational change in purposes, policies, and methods in a particular instance, particularly when cast in ideological terms:

> It seems clear these macroscopic developments [affecting societal consciousness] provided a cultural milieu that served to sensitize the staff to problems of racism, poverty, and institutional malfunction and to create a predisposition to experiment with new forms of service delivery including client advocacy and community action. Moreover, it seems likely that the

widespread criticism of organizations for their unresponsive and irrelevant policies provoked the staff of FCS [the agency, i.e., the social orga-
nization] to examine not only their own programs but also those of other
agencies. This *ideological* climate seems to have been at least a necessary
foundation for the transformation observed although it is insufficient as a
consideration for change (1972, p. 246, emphasis supplied).

The cultural milieu of which Patti and Resnick speak, and the ideological
climate which they describe, may or may not be sufficient to induce organizational change, but they do connote the behavioral expectations which they can
generate, and the ethics they may inspire. In any event, as ethical responsibility
the expectations persist.

The Ethical Responsibility of Social Organizations

There are other ethical responsibilities which may be attributed to social
organizations as organizations, but perhaps those which have been discussed
will suffice to indicate that, although it is invariably people who will be looked
to for the implementation of those responsibilities, it is to the social organization as an institutional entity that these responsibilities will be ascribed. A
receptionist may be offensive, a secretary may be officious, a social caseworker
may be negligent, a statistician may lie, an administrator may exploit subordinates. To each may be attributed ethical responsibility of one kind or another in
relation to the occupational functions they perform in the organization, but to
all of them collectively may be attributed an order and range of ethical responsibilities which are clearly related to the organization's mission and function in
the community and society. Their behavior in their organizational capacity will
occasion the judgment that, "In this kind of organization, this is the way the
employee is expected to act," or, "That kind of conduct is not fitting in such an
organization." Whatever it is that the organization is supposed to do or represent institutionally, all of its personnel are expected to reflect in their behavior
in their organizational capacity.

Whether addressed to individual persons, or to other organizations, or to the
community and society at large, the ethical responsibility of the social organization is meant for human beings—how they are treated, how they are served,
how they are accounted to, how their interests are represented.

The operation of the organization may be guided by *scientism* or it may be
guided by *humanism*:

By scientism we refer to the approach which assumes that any problem
can be reduced logically to definable and measurable parts and that a
single best solution can be found to maximize the organization's goal or
objective. . . . Such an approach emphasizes a technical, task-oriented

approach to problems, with conviction that the most efficient option must override less important things, even including the individual preferences . . . [or] happiness of participants. . . . By the term humanism we refer to a contracting approach to organizational issues which defines them as basically human concerns (Holland, 1978, pp. 23-24).

Organizational ethics is clearly a function of human concerns, with responsibility for them being lodged in human beings who represent the interests and responsibility of the organization to which organizational ethics may be ascribed. However, a scientific perspective may be required to understand organizational ethics sufficiently and to make it operational.

REFERENCES

Addams, Jane. *Democracy and Social Ethics,* Ann Firor Scott, ed. (Cambridge, Mass.: Harvard University Press, 1964). First published in 1907.

Du Noüy, Pierre Lecomte. *Between Knowing and Believing,* Trans. Mary Lecomte Du Noüy (New York: David McKay Co., 1966).

Etzioni, Amitai. *Modern Organizations* (Englewood Cliffs, N.J.: Prentice-Hall, 1964).

Holland, Thomas P. "Scientism and Humanism in Management Decision-Making," *Journal of Applied Social Sciences,* 2 (1978), 23-32.

Kaplan, Abraham. *The New World of Philosophy* (New York: Vintage Books, 1961).

Miller, David. *Social Justice* (Oxford: Clarendon Press, 1976).

Patti, Rino J. and Resnick, Herman. "The Dynamics of Agency Change," *Social Casework,* 53 (1972), 243-55.

Rawls, John. *A Theory of Justice* (Cambridge, Mass.: Harvard University Press, 1971).

Ross, Edward Alsworth. *Social Control: A Survey of the Foundations of Order* (Cleveland, Ohio: The Press of Case Western Reserve University, 1969). First published in 1901.

Simon, Herbert, Smithburg, Donald W., and Thompson, Victor A. *Public Administration* (New York: Alfred A. Knopf, 1958).

Vinter, Robert D. "New Evidence for Restructuring Group Services," in *New Perspectives on Services to Groups: Theory, Organization, Practice* (New York: National Association of Social Workers, 1961), 48-69.

IV. ADMINISTRATIVE ETHICS
FOR NON-ADMINISTRATIVE STAFF

I have said that the ethics of social work administration is a function of the purposes served by social organizations; of the relationships in and of social organizations which are associated with those purposes; of the responsibilities of organization personnel—both paid and volunteer—which are related to those purposes; and of the societal, organizational, and occupational norms and expectations by which evaluations of both organizations and their personnel are guided. Robert Presthus conceives of organizations in terms quite compatible with this conception of administrative ethics in social organizations, for he defines them as "'miniature societies' in which the dominant values of society are inculcated and sought in a more structured, spatially restricted context" (1962, p. vii). Presthus, in his book, discusses "the influence of social values and bureacratic structure upon members of the big organizations that pervade our society," and "the patterns of individual accommodations that occur in the bureaucratic milieu" (p. 3). Naturally enough, Presthus emphasizes the pervasive influence that contemporary organizations have on individual and group behavior, especially through the use of rewards, sanctions, and other inducements. However, ethics may be viewed as a means of coping with organizational influences and inducements as well as a means of accommodating them.

Ethics and Organizational Control

The ethics of social work administration includes obligations in and to social organizations; to the various persons with whom relationships and contacts are generated by the purposes and functions of the organizations; and to the various persons who are affected by them. On the other hand, the occupational ethics by which the activities of organization personnel may be guided and influenced often represents means for contending with organizational demands.

As much as social organizations control and coordinate non-administrative personnel—which is to say that as much as the administrators of social organizations do or try to control and coordinate the efforts and activities of all organization personnel, including those who do not carry administrative responsibility as such—it is part and parcel of the ethical responsibility of those personnel to *be* controlled and coordinated. They are organization men and women not only in the sociological sense and in the sociopsychological sense explicated by William Whyte in *The Organization Man* (1956), but also in the ethical sense. As employees of social organizations, non-administrative as well as administrative personnel owe ethical duties to those social organizations. Perhaps as precautionary measures, social organizations, like organizations in general, use a variety of means to control and coordinate the efforts and activities of all personnel, including those who are not charged with administrative responsibility.

March and Simon, in analyzing studies of organizations by Merton, Selznick, and Gouldner, found that all three employed "as the basic independent variable some form of organization or organizational procedure designed to control the activities of the organization members" (1958, p. 37). They considered these procedures to be based primarily on what they described as the "machine" model of human behavior, although they were obviously aware of the fact that organization theorists and practitioners have more recently emphasized a more humanistic approach to the administration of organizations. Even this emphasis may not be all it is cracked up to be, for it may merely substitute one form of control for another, less out of a humanitarian concern for employees and others perhaps than out of concern about the successful management—or control—of organizations. There is not much reason to believe that social organizations are less affected by the latter concern than profit-making and industrial organizations, for even in them very often the maintenance and preservation of the organization, and the control of its personnel, are of greater concern to its administrators than the social purposes—social service, for example—for which the organization presumably exists.

Coordination, a critical managerial and administrative function in social organizations, is another form of organizational control which has its counterpart in the ethics of social work administration. That is, as with organizational control in general, staff members employed by a social organization are under the moral obligation to the social organization, and under the constraints of occupational ethics when subject to a code of professional ethics, to facilitate efforts at organizational coordination. In Simon's words,

> Group behavior requires not only the adoption of correct decisions, but also the adoption by all members of the same decisions. . . . Writers on the political and legal aspects of authority have emphasized that a primary function of organization is to enforce the conformity of the individual to norms laid down by the group, or by its authority-wielding members. . . . When exercising authority, the superior does not seek to convince the subordinate, but only to obtain his acquiescence (1957, pp. 10-11).

That is the administrative point of view. Ethically, it is incumbent upon subordinates to acquiesce. But, like other requirements of the ethics of social work administration, this requirement is never absolute. To ignore it is not the same as being ethical, but this does not mean that there are never conditions under which it may be, and perhaps must be, ignored. Simon provides a clue to the mutuality of obligations between organization and staff member, and to a determinant of the latter's ethical responsibility and its operation—*if* it is to operate:

> The term *organization* refers to the complex pattern of communications and other relations in a group of human beings. This pattern provides to each member of the group much of the information, assumptions, goals, and attitudes that enter into his decisions, and provides him with a set of stable and comprehensible expectations as to what the other members of the group are doing and how they would react to what he says and does (p. xvi).

What Simon adds to this observation—which applies as much to non-administrative personnel as it does to the administrators toward whom Simon is primarily oriented—makes quite evident its ethical connotations, for he has the administrator put to himself the following question: "What do the choices I have made . . . show about my values and the values that others in the organization impute to me?" (p. xvii) The values behind the staff member's choices and actions represent the ethics by which the choices and actions are guided, or so they appear to others to be.

The purposes, functions, operations, and relationships of social organizations shape the ethical responsibilities of all organization personnel, although these responsibilities vary according to the status of the personnel—whether volunteer or paid, and whether or not occupationally identified in their capacity in the organization. These responsibilities also vary according to the functional capacity of personnel in the organization. In addition to the ethical responsibilities shared by all personnel in the organization, all also carry particular ethical responsibilities as associated with the occupations with which they are identified, and as associated with or attributable to their assignments and job descriptions.

Sources of Ethical Responsibility in Social Organizations

The responsibilities of volunteers—board members, for example—derive from their position as trustees of the community, and as representatives of the interests of the community from which the organization acquires its sanction to operate. Their responsibilities derive also from their position as policy-makers and monitors of the social services and functions which the organization and its personnel perform. The first position requires an accounting to the community, and the second position requires an accounting to the organization's clientele and other beneficiaries of the organization's functions and services. An accounting is due as well to others who may be affected by those functions and services, or who otherwise share a stake in what the organization is and does.

Paid personnel may or may not have specifically assigned or ascribed administrative responsibilities. When they do, they are administrators and therefore are accountable for whatever may constitute the ethics of social work administration. This does not mean that administrative ethics is not also a responsibility of staff members of social organizations who do not carry specifically assigned administrative responsibilities.

In a way, the title of this chapter is a contradiction since nobody in a social organization does not carry administrative responsibility. On the other hand, some of the organization's paid personnel have explicitly defined administrative responsibility, and thus share the responsibility for administering the organization. Others to whom administrative responsibility may be ascribed carry administrative responsibility only in the sense that whatever they do in the organization and for the organization makes incumbent upon them certain administrative responsibilities. That is, such administrative responsibilities as may be attributed to them are a consequence of the non-administrative work to which they are assigned in the organization. In this sense, administration is everybody's business in the organization because whatever anyone in the organization does affects and is affected by its administrative structure, processes, and procedures. Everyone in the organization has an administrative accounting to make for what is or is not done in the implementation of organizational responsibility and purposes, and in dealing with the administrative relationships and instrumentalities required to carry them out.

I have already considered that aspect of this observation which is associated with the community's sanction and support of the purposes and functions of social organizations. Whatever the norms and values of the community and society which come to represent expectations for the organization because of whatever it is the organization is formally or informally sanctioned to do, those norms and values become commitments for all of the organization's personnel—commitments which serve as guides to their conduct in, and on behalf of, the organization. In addition, however, all organization staff members carry responsibilities of an ethical as well as functional nature in relation to the organization's administrators, administrative structure, administrative processes, and administrative procedures.

Ethics as Intended Conduct

Ethical conduct is intended conduct. Administrative ethics is also intentional, however incidental administrative responsibility is to the assignments of organization staff members. Staff members, including non-administrative staff members, are supposed to be aware of what it is ethically incumbent upon them to do in their various organizational capacities, including that which is done in response to their share of administrative responsibility. This seems to be the intent of the Parsonian frame of reference as Calvin J. Larson sees it:

> Action as opposed to behavior is viewed essentially as the intervention of the element of decision-making . . . between stimulus and response. . . . A situation may be thought of as a stage, an arena, or a setting in which an actor is obliged to decide between alternative roles to play (1977, p. 132).

The element of decision-making is as critical in the fulfillment of ethical responsibility in relation to the administration of social organizations as it is in the fulfillment of administrative responsibilities as such.[1] Before staff members take any action, they are obliged to determine the course of action most responsive to the values to which they are ethically committed in their contention with situations charged with administrative as well as other functional considerations. It is not enough for staff members to do their duty as their particular occupational roles are defined. They are also ethically responsible to consider the administrative impact of their actions as well as the relationship to their occupational roles of the organization's administrative structure, processes, policies, and procedures. This applies to typist, social caseworker, nurse, and anyone else with an organizational role to play, whether assigned administrative responsibility as such or not.

Ethical Responsibility of Non-Administrative Staff: The Case of the Social Worker

Social workers who are not employed in a social organization to perform administrative roles can serve to illustrate the import of these observations. In some degree, what is said about social workers is applicable to other personnel who are employed to perform other occupational functions, with the chief difference being that the latter are subject to whatever ethical injunctions are applicable to their particular occupational functions. If they are members of occupations for which ethics has been codified, as it has been for social workers, then they may be assumed to be guided by the codes of ethics of the occupations to which they belong, and subject to the constraints and enforcement of those codes.

A reasonable starting point, as far as social workers are concerned, is the

---

[1]"Administration is ordinarily discussed as the art of 'getting things done.' Emphasis is placed upon processes and methods for insuring incisive action. Principles are set forth for securing concerted action . . . Not very much attention is paid to the choice which prefaces all action—to the determining of what is to be done rather than to the actual doing. . . .

"Although any practical activity involves both 'deciding' and 'doing,' it has not commonly been recognized that a theory of administration should be concerned with the process of decision as well as with the processes of action. . . . The task of 'deciding' pervades the entire administrative organization quite as much as the task of 'doing'—indeed, it is integrally tied up with the latter. A general theory of administration must include principles of organization that will insure correct decision-making, just as it must include principles that will insure effective action" (Simon, 1957, p. 1).

codification of the principles of ethical practice in relation to employers and employing organizations in the Code of Ethics of the National Association of Social Workers, adopted by the Association's Delegate Assembly in 1979 (the full text of which is given in the Appendix of this book).

IV L. *Commitment to Employing Organization*
The social worker should adhere to commitments made to the employing organization.

1. The social worker should work to improve the employing agency's policies and procedures, and the efficiency and effectiveness of its services.
2. The social worker should not accept employment or arrange student field placement in an organization which is currently under public sanction by NASW for violating personnel standards or imposing limitations on, or penalties for, professional actions on behalf of clients.
3. The social worker should act to prevent and eliminate discrimination in the employing organization's work assignments and in its employment policies and practices.
4. The social worker should use with scrupulous regard, and only for the purpose for which they are intended, the resources of the employing organization (1979).

These four principles of ethical practice, designed to guide the conduct of social workers in relation to employers and employing organizations, along with the overarching principle which is cited to introduce the four principles, reflect and suggest the scope of ethical responsibility assignable to social work staff members as their share of responsibility for the ethics of social work administration. They stem from the major premise that, though social workers are expected to fulfill the professional responsibilities which they are employed to perform in relation to clients, they also incur ethical responsibility in relation to the employing organization and its administration. This does not mean, however, that their ethical responsibility to the employing organization is boundless. Loyalty and devotion to the employing organization, like loyalty and devotion to the clients that social workers are employed to serve as an integral element in the employment arrangement,[2] is neither absolute nor infinite.

Nevertheless, the very acceptance of employment in a social organization

---

[2]"II. *The Social Worker's Ethical Responsibility to Clients*
F. *Primacy of Clients' Interests*
The Social Worker's Primary Responsibility Is to Clients.
1. The social worker should serve clients with devotion, loyalty, determination, and the maximum application of professional skill and competence" (1979).

constitutes in itself a promise of loyalty to the organization and devotion to its purposes and functions, particularly but not exclusively those to which the social worker has a direct or indirect operational relationship. This applies to whatever understanding both social worker and organization leadership have of the responsibilities to be carried by the social worker on behalf of the organization, and the organization's responsibility to the social worker.

The employer-employee relationship which links organization and social worker is an administrative relationship. That is, it is a relationship designed and created to help facilitate the implementation of the organization's policies, and the fulfillment of its purposes. In the terms of that relationship, the assumption is made, or attributable to both parties, that whatever the administrative arrangements for carrying out the work of the organization, and for making possible the fulfillment of the social worker's assigned responsibilities, both parties will live by them and make them operational.

These arrangements which are usually governed by the organization's personnel practices and administrative procedures, include terms of employment, like salary to be paid the social worker; the social worker's times on and off the job; procedures to be followed and equipment to be made available in the performance of the social worker's functions; budgets within the framework of which services are to be rendered the organization's clients or programs provided for the organization's constituents; procedures for projecting budgets and for accounting for expenditures; and so on. For each of these arrangements, ethical responsibilities are implied for both the social worker and the organization. The arrangements define the substance of personnel practices and administrative procedures. The ethics defines the values by which their implementation is guided and evaluated.

Every staff member has the ethical responsibility to spend wisely, and for the purpose intended, the money of the organization which has been allocated to an activity, a service, a program, or a procedure for which the staff member has assigned responsibility or a share of concern. The staff member also has the ethical responsibility to anticipate accurately and realistically the cost of the activity, the service, the program, or the procedure—to the extent that the staff member shares responsibility for such projections—in the interest of sound organizational budgeting, but primarily in the interest of responsiveness to a moral obligation. The breadth of the responsibility to provide administrators with the information they need for various purposes including budgeting is suggested by David F. Gillespie.

> Administrative responsibilities revolve around and depend upon information. Planning, coordinating, assembling and allocating resources, supervising, evaluating, policy setting, and the rest are more or less effective depending upon the quality of information available (1977, pp. 406-407).

Such dependency in any occupational relationship, like that between staff members and administrators of social organizations, is one of the foundations of occupational ethics in general, and of the administrative ethics of non-administrative organization staff. Whatever procedures have been defined for accomplishing the work of the social organization, non-administrative staff members are obliged to follow, whether those procedures affect access to the secretarial pool, or the requisition and acquisition of supplies, or whatever. They are accountable also for their role in procedures for their own supervision and for evaluating their job performance and their contributions to the performance by the organization as a whole of its social and administrative functions. All of these are fundamental managerial necessities but they are also ethical ones. Their importance lies not only in their utility for making it possible for all staff to play their appropriate roles, but also in their symbolization of the ethical responsibility shared by non-administrative staff members as participants in the organization's administrative structure. Whatever they do in their organizational capacity must be ultimately, if not also immediately, related to the organization's goals, and the effectiveness and efficiency with which those goals are achieved. As Etzioni has put it:

> The goals of organizations . . . set down guide lines for organizational activity. . . . Moreover, goals serve as standards by which members of an organization and outsiders can assess the success of the organization— i.e., its effectiveness and efficiency. . . . An organizational goal is a desired state of affairs which the organization attempts to realize. . . . The actual *effectiveness* of a specific organization is determined by the degree to which it realizes its goals. The *efficiency* of an organization is measured by the amount of resources used to produce a unit of output. Output is usually closely related to, but not identical with, the organizational goals. . . . Efficiency increases as the costs (resources used) decrease. . . . Efficiency and effectiveness [do not always] go hand in hand (1964, pp. 5-9).

Social workers who are not assigned specific administrative responsibilities but, rather, perform service and program functions of one kind or another, like counseling clients or leading activity groups, are accountable for administrative ethics primarily as it is a function of the relationship between the social workers and the organization, and between the social workers and the organization's administrators at all levels. Since organizations *as* organizations cannot relate to persons, or persons to organizations, except through organizational representatives, the ethics of social work administration for non-administrative staff members affects the relationship between those staff members and all of the organization's administrators. Included among the latter are the chief executive and all sub-executives, department heads, supervisors—all administrative personnel to whom the staff members are in any way accountable for the performance of their functions. Also included are those to whom they must relate or with whom they must deal in the performance of their functions, or simply those whom their behavior in their organizational capacity affects. But, again, these are all two-way streets.

Non-administrative staff members also have ethical responsibility to the collectivity of administrators as representatives of the organization and its interests in general. All of the ethical duties owed to employers and employing organizations apply both as organizational obligations and as obligations to colleagues.

The conscientious and purposeful use of organizational resources is almost a self-evident ethical requirement—I say almost because it is so frequently violated, and with virtual communal sanction at that. Still, organization funds, materials, and all of the other resources placed at the disposal of non-administrative staff members are not personal assets, regardless of the autonomy they may enjoy in the organization. They are assets held in trust for the community and the society unless and until used for the purposes for which they are meant. It is an ethical imperative that they be used economically and productively.

Policy Conflicts for Social Workers

Other ethical responsibilities are not so self-evident. For many non-administrative staff members they are even controversial. Adherence to commitments made to the employing organization by the social worker, for example, implies the honoring of all organization policies, the assumption being that none violates existing laws or ethical principles, or the terms of employment between the social worker and the organization. If a social organization enunciates eligibility requirements—whether via legislative or charter-like conditions to be met, for example, for financial assistance or marital counseling—it is incumbent on staff members to apply those requirements when serving the organization's clientele, whether the staff members agree with them or not. It is not ethical for staff members to negotiate policy differences with the organization's clients, or to contend with them by violating or obstructing policies which are in effect. On the other hand, it is also incumbent on staff members to provide whatever clients are eligible for even if administrators disapprove.

Not all social organizations are so extensively staffed or hierarchically ordered as to involve essentially non-administrative personnel in the kinds of intricate relationships and exposures that make issues of this type so common. Some organizations are small in fact, small enough to require no more than one or two levels of administrative organization and authority. And there are some organizations that are limited to one—the so-called one-man or one-woman agencies where a single staff member carries all service and all administrative responsibilities. Small family service agencies in small communities exist in appreciable number in the United States and Canada. In such agencies, conflicts in relation to organization policy are less likely to arise except as they are discussed in meetings of boards of directors.

Conflicts that non-administrative personnel—and often lower-level administrative staff—experience in relation to organization policies which they find it difficult or distasteful to abide by, are usually conflicts with administrators. That administrators are sensitive to the prospect of such conflicts, and the prospect of staff deviation which may be too obscured or ambiguous to become a basis for disciplinary action, is indicated by the preoccupation in social organizations as well as business and industrial organizations with processes of control and compliance.

The larger the organization, the greater the likelihood of anonymity for non-administrative personnel. The greater, therefore, the inclination to deviate from expectations associated with their relationship to the organization as a whole, and to their administrative colleagues. Collusion with clients in the infringement of organization policies is easier, and often more inspired, when it connotes for staff members primacy of clients' interests and a contribution to social justice, as when the policy violated impresses staff members as inherently unjust. Nevertheless, from the point of view of administrative ethics, such collusion is unethical even if staff members consider it justifiable in relation to the ethical responsibility they feel they have towards clients. The dilemma for them is simply that they may not be able to accommodate both responsibilities at the same time, and to accommodate one may be to violate another. Perhaps it is this type of dilemma that moved Paul Kurzman to write:

> The rules and regulations that practitioners [in large-scale social welfare institutions] so frequently lament as burdensome and obstructive tend to meet certain survival needs of the organization. . . . In a large-scale organization, decisions are based upon two kinds of premises: factual and valuational . . . the stability of the organization is in part dependent on maintaining a balance between the two. It would upset the organization's stability if there were no rules . . . because the institution has to survive in a valuational world. . . . What rules and regulations do is attempt to reduce the valuational component (1977, pp. 422-423).

For social workers, the valuational component is contained both in the ethics of social work practice with clients, and in the ethics of social work administration as it affects social workers who work with clients but are not assigned specific and direct administrative responsibilities. Very often, social workers feel themselves at odds with organization administrators over issues of policy which the social workers regard as antithetical to the interests of clients. Social workers often insist that it is precisely in clients' interests that the organization exists in the first place. They often insist that it is clients' interests that social workers are supposed to represent, both as staff members in the organization and as members of the social work profession. These responses on the part of social workers tend to make them actual though invisible adversaries of the administrators.

Organizational Maintenance Versus Organizational Effectiveness

The aim of effective and economical implementation of the organization's purposes usually contributes to the motivation of administrators to control employees and induce their compliance with organizational policies and procedures. Such motivation is often also influenced by their zeal for the maintenance and preservation of the organization whether or not its survival correlates well with its functional effectiveness. This was one of the "secrets" of organizations that Gouldner "revealed";

> According to the conventional view of welfare agencies, these groups exist in order to satisfy a community need or to solve a community problem. Nominally, welfare agencies are supposed to be instrumental devices, tools that the community creates to solve its problems. It is certainly no dark secret, however, but perhaps more akin to an open secret, that agencies and their programs come to be regarded by their staff as valuable *in their own right,* and that they seek to survive regardless of the effectiveness with which they solve the community's problems (1963, p. 164).

Since the community's problems with which welfare agencies deal include the problems of clients which social workers attend to, these problems are also affected by this illuminated secret. This makes especially ironical Gouldner's observation that "one of the groups which the welfare agencies help, and for whom they provide basic gratifications, are the social workers themselves" (p. 162). To the extent that this is true, social workers are just as apt as agency administrators to put a high priority on organizational survival and maintenance, if necessary at the expense of clients and the services that the agency is committed to provide to them. But it is not always true. For many social workers this does not constitute a personal priority sufficient to avoid a feeling of conflict as between agency interest and client interest. Therefore, for example, if in the interest of its own solvency it is the policy of a hospital for a social worker to encourage patients to remain in the hospital or to undergo surgery when neither may be in the patients' best interests, and the social worker has good and sufficient reason to know as much in a particular case, the social worker may not so easily and readily conform to institutional demand. Responsibility to client may override responsibility to hospital and inspire the social worker to evade the hospital's policy, and in so doing to offend the ethical principle of adhering to commitments to the employing organization. (The ethics of agency policies also merits inquiry.)

Adherence to the policies of a social organization does not mean exemption from the responsibility to change the policies—or anything else in the organization for that matter—when they intrude on the achievement of the organization's program and service goals, particularly when the intrusion adversely affects the organization's clientele and its prospective clientele. But, short of manifestly unethical organization policies and practices, the media for such change are not the organization's clients as manipulated by staff members, although clients may be provided with such guidance as they may require and enlist regarding the channels for policy change at their disposal, and such assistance as they may require to afford them access to those channels. Such help is part and parcel of a social worker's professional function with organization clients, the function that a social worker is presumably engaged by the organization to perform.

On the other hand, it is as much the social worker's moral obligation—it is as much an ethical responsibility—to assist the organization in reconsidering its policies and procedures, as it is to abide by those policies and procedures. And it is the social worker's moral obligation to help the organization improve its service to its client just as much as it is to serve clients with maximum loyalty, devotion, and competence. The social worker's relationship to the employing organization, and responsibility in and to it, like the social worker's relationship and responsibility to clients, is the basis for the ethical responsibility ascribed to the social worker.

In considering the social worker's approach to organizational change and the factors contributing to resistance to change, Rino J. Patti makes the following assumptions:

> That the practitioner is attempting in good faith to effect change in the organization's policies, programs, or procedures in order that it may be a more effective instrument for the delivery of social services . . . that the change agent is competent and responsible in the performance of his professional role and that his involvement in the change effort is not intended to divert attention from or displace responsibility for his own personal or professional inadequacies . . . [and] that he has conscientiously attempted to formulate his proposal on the basis of the best and most complete information available to him . . . Unless these conditions have been met, the resistance the administrative subordinate encounters may be attributable more to him than the organization he seeks to change (1974, p. 369).

Ethics Versus Competence in Relation to Policy Change

It is not merely good will that is required for non-administrative as well as administrative organizational personnel to act on their ethical responsibility to both client and organization, but also competence. It is not that competence is a measure of administrative ethics; only that for the implementation of ethical responsibility competence may be required.[3]

The necessary competence provided for, the ethical responsibility of non-administrative personnel remains to do whatever needs doing, through legitimate organizational channels, to change those policies and procedures that militate against the achievement of the employing organization's basic purposes; or that do not conduce maximally to meeting the needs of the organization's clientele; or that in any way limit the access of clientele to services related to those needs. For social workers, this may be interpreted both as professional responsibility and as organizational responsibility, for it represents for social workers their moral obligations as members of the social work profession and as employees of the organization for which they are working as social workers.

The reaches of this statement are implicit in the following comment by Brenda McGowan:

> One of the distinguishing characteristics of all professionals is that they are bound by ethical codes prescribing a service ideal in which client interests are expected to come before personal interests. Although service organizations are also expected to benefit their clients, they are not bound [I read this as likely or liable to. C.S.L.] to place individual client need above organizational interest; and as Gouldner has suggested, one of the best kept secrets of service organizations is that the primary goal is often that of organizational self-maintenance (1978, p. 158).

McGowan goes on to specify a problem illustrative of the kind of action which might be required of non-administrative social workers and the issue in ethics it can pose.

---

[3]Compare the following comments on the issue of professional competence as it affects the social worker's ethical responsibility to clients: "Social work ethics . . . affects the substance of the social worker's technical competence as a social worker less than the manner in which that competence is applied in a client's behalf. A modicum of competence must be assumed before ethical issues can be contended with because the ethical component of social work practice implies choice on the social worker's part and the capacity to exercise it. . . . The existence or nonexistence of social work competence . . . can itself be conceived of as an ethical issue" (Levy, 1976, p. 109). "Competence is charged with a moral dimension in the sense that the social worker is expected to feel obliged to be specifically equipped to perform the specific function he undertakes as well as to undertake social work service in the first place" (p. 117).

Organizational goals often have a strong social control component . . .
An overemphasis on results may lead to a selection of clients who are
most likely to succeed rather than provision of services to those most in
need . . . *Creaming* . . . effective results can often be achieved through
questionable means that raise ethical dilemmas for the professional (p.
159).

Client Versus Organization

How far do social workers—or other non-administrative organization employees—go in choosing a course of action which is more responsive to ethical
responsibility to clients than to the employing organization? What if social
workers exhaust the legitimate channels of the organization at their disposal and
still fail to effect the change sought in clients' behalf? Up to this point their
actions may be assumed to be ethical since they fit within the framework of
professional responsibility to both clients and organization. Beyond that, one or
the other must succumb. Whichever does succumb represents a violation of
ethical responsibility. On the other hand, the ethics of social work administration may require or necessitate precisely that kind of violation—at least as a
social worker may see it. It then becomes a matter of demonstrating that
the deviation was justified on the grounds of superseding values. But it is a
deviation.

A rather pervasive manifestation of this effect in a number of professions,
and in businesses and industries as well as government agencies in which those
professions operate, is what has been described as "whistle-blowing" for which
various codes of ethics make rather protective provisions.[4] The opportunities for
social workers in social organizations to "blow the whistle" may appear to be
more limited than they are for scientists and engineers—and, perhaps, for the
"deep throats" of government—but they do exist. Social workers may know
about discriminatory and even fraudulent practices in their employing organizations—practices that hurt or deprive clients in one way or another, or practices
insufficiently responsive to the accountability of the organizations to their community, their contributors, or to others—but be entirely unsuccessful in their
attempts to change those practices. The first obligation, of course, is to try as
much as possible to do something about those practices. Whether a social
worker goes public with information about them is a decision not to be taken
lightly, even in a self-righteous acknowledgement of the obligation to clients,

---

[4]See, for example, the "Agenda Book for the Workshop on Professional Ethics: The Role of
Scientific and Engineering Societies," The Professional Ethics Project of the American Association
for the Advancement of Science, November 15-16, 1979, for samples of principles and cases. See
also Nader, Petkas, and Blackwell (1972).

to community, or to society. It is the organization that the social worker works for, directly and specifically, not clients, the community, or society.

Even the social worker's relationships to clients are directed and dictated by the employment arrangement with the organization. Nevertheless, these also represent moral obligations and ethical requirements. The ultimate question for the social worker is the degree of priority to accord these and other obligations. The discretion of the social worker in contending with them must be scrupulously and discreetly employed. The choice must be based upon the seriousness and the consequences of the organization's failing; the relationship of the failing to the organization's obligations to others; and the relationship and responsibility of the social worker to both. Whistle-blowing is not always justifiable, but it is often necessary in the interest of fairness and justice, and in the interest of institutional responsibility. Whatever it is that the social worker may offer in justification of the act after the fact—for example, in an adjudication of a complaint or a grievance brought under the Code of Ethics of the social work profession—the social worker should carefully consider before the act.

In these cases it is not the principles of ethical practice or conduct that are being negotiated or renegotiated. The contention with the ethical issues in each case is not directed toward the discovery of the best ethical alternative or the most apt ethical principle. It is rather—and this applies to both adjudication and choices of action—to determine on the basis of all of the facts in each case, and all of the considerations relevant to it—including the various ethical responsibilities of the social worker—which principles of ethics to employ and which *not* to employ. This kind of ethical judgment necessarily leads to the possibility—not the inevitability—of adverse or uncomfortable consequences for the social worker. What this kind of choice indicates is that some things—honesty, for example, or the rights and needs of clients—are so valued that even clearly prescribed and defined responsibilities and commitments are abrogated. The social worker then throws himself or herself at the mercy of the court, as it were; nor can the defense for the vagary—since in ethical terms, that is what it is—be at the level of defense for a defendant who was charged with the murder of his parents and then pleaded for mercy because he was an orphan. The social worker's grounds must be more substantial than that.

Loyalty—Quo Vadis

Similar considerations affect other failures to live up to commitments to an organization, failures not so readily justified regardless of an employee's good will and good intentions. Does the social worker, for example, reveal the secrets of the employing organization in the zeal to correct or prevent an injustice or organizational hanky-panky? The moralist may be inclined to say, of course. On the other hand, that is tantamount to admitting that the social worker is free to betray confidences acquired because, and in the course, of employment. Again, the "cause" may be regarded as transcending the ethical responsibility to the employing organization. Nevertheless, the justification must be compelling, just as it would be expected to be in the relationship of the social worker to clients.

Many of the principles of ethical practice which apply to the social worker's relationship to clients, in fact, would appear to be applicable to the social worker's relationship to the employing organization, since the relationship to the employing organization in many ways is analogous to the relationship to clients. If this seems to be a contradiction, in light of the social worker's relationship to clients *in* the organization, one should remember that the relationship to clients exists *because* of the employment in and by the organization, and on its behalf.

Though this may limit the social worker who is moved to action in the organization because of disservice or insufficient service to clients—even aggressive action—it can also have an enabling effect. Since the social worker is employed by the organization to provide service to clients, with all of the applicable conventions of professional service—short of grossly destructive and erratic acts and manifestly unprofessional conduct—it should be possible for the social worker to validate an attempt to change an organization policy or procedure in the interests of clients, precisely on the basis that it is those interests which the social worker has been employed by the organization to represent and serve. That is inside the organization. Going outside the organization to represent and serve the interests of clients when all else fails would no doubt require a strong case—and a strong social worker.

Although I have been discussing the ethical responsibility of the non-administrative employee to the social organization as a whole, that responsibility affects primarily the relationship of the employee to the organization's administrative personnel. As far as the social worker is concerned, therefore, the provisions in the NASW Code of Ethics concerning the social worker's ethical responsibility to colleagues would be applicable. Some of those provisions coincide with the provisions in the Code affecting the employer and employing organization. The expectation is that the employee will treat the administrators of the organization with respect, courtesy, fairness, and good faith; that the employee will respect confidences which administrators share; that the employee will treat with respect, and represent accurately and fairly, the qualifications, views, and findings of administrators, and use appropriate channels to express judgments on these matters.

On the other hand, the employee is also obliged, as the Code has it, to "take adequate measures to discourage, prevent, expose, and correct the unethical conduct of colleagues," as well as "defend and assist colleagues unjustly charged with unethical conduct" (1979, Preamble).

Non-administrative personnel may not be assigned administrative responsibility as such, but the ethics of social work administration demands of them much that has consequences for the social organizations in which, and by which, they are employed, and for those who have anything to do with them.

REFERENCES

Etzioni, Amitai. *Modern Organizations* (Englewood Cliffs, N.J.: Prentice-Hall, 1964).

Gillespie, David F. "Discovering and Describing Organizational Goal Conflict," *Administration in Social Work,* 1 (1977), 395-408.

Gouldner, Alvin W. "The Secrets of Organizations," *The Social Welfare Forum 1963* (New York: Columbia University Press, 1963), 161-177.

Kurzman, Paul A. "Rules and Regulations in Large-Scale Organizations: A Theoretical Approach to the Problem," *Administration in Social Work,* 1 (1977), 421-431.

Larson, Calvin J. *Major Themes in Social Theory* (2nd Ed.; New York: David McKay Co., 1977).

Levy, Charles S. *Social Work Ethics* (New York: Human Sciences Press, 1976).

March, James G. and Simon, Herbert A. *Organizations* (New York: John Wiley and Sons, 1958).

McGowan, Brenda G. "Strategies in Bureaucracies," in Judith S. Mearig and associates, *Working for Children: Ethical Issues Beyond Professional Guidelines* (San Francisco: Jossey-Bass Publishers, 1978), Chapter 9.

Nader, Ralph, Petkas, Peter J., and Blackwell, Kate, Eds. *Whistle Blowing* (New York: Grossman, 1972).

National Association of Social Workers. Code of Ethics, adopted by the NASW Delegate Assembly, November 18, 1979 (see Appendix).

Patti, Rino J. "Organizational Resistance and Change: The View from Below," *Social Service Review,* 48 (1974), 367-383.

Presthus, Robert. *The Organizational Society: An Analysis and a Theory* (New York: Vintage Books, 1962).

Simon, Herbert A. *Administrative Behavior: A Study of Decision-Making Process in Administrative Organization* (2nd ed.; New York: The Free Press, 1957).

Whyte, William H., Jr. *The Organization Man* (New York: Simon and Schuster, 1956).

V. THE EXECUTIVE

Except for such constraints on the power of a social organization executive as the organization's governing board or other controlling body is authorized and willing to use—and, all too often, the board is disinclined or reluctant to impose such constraints—the executive is, in many ways, invested with virtually unlimited power over many things and persons. The larger and more bureaucratic the organization, and the more autonomous the executive, the greater the opportunity to exploit or abuse such power with relative impunity. The smaller the organization, on the other hand, the more direct and unsettling the experience for victims of such exploitation and abuse, and the more personal the effects may be or may feel.

Not that there are no other controls, external or internal, over executive action. Forces in the community may be in operation to restrain the executive's use of the power at his or her disposal. And there are also internal media of control at the disposal of organization members and personnel—not all of which are normative, legal, or ethical—through which executives may receive their come-uppance, if not more devastating and enduring consequences. Many an organization executive has been organizationally and vocationally destroyed by vindictive board or staff members, and by alignments between and among them; and not always with cause. Executives do have their quota of vulnerabilities which others in the organization may see fit to exploit, and this they sometimes do.

The ethics of social work administration applicable to the non-administrative personnel of a social organization, which was considered in Chapter Four and which is at least equally applicable to subordinate administrative personnel, is in part designed or calculated to prevent or avoid the abuses of power—especially informally accrued power—by which executives can be readily victimized by others. Confrontations between executives and others in organizations which descend to this level are of course symptomatic of fundamental organizational problems. Such problems often have consequences, not only for organization members and personnel, but also for organization clients. The treatment of clients and the services made available to them are often adversely affected as a result. But confrontations need not start or remain at so primitive a level to validate principles of ethical conduct relevant to relationships between executives and others inside and outside of the organization.

Executive Power and Vulnerability

As vulnerable as executives of social organizations may be to derogation, defamation, disparagement, and undermining by others, they do have access to considerable power over the fate, the destiny, the opportunities, and the comfort of others. And yet, they may be the least autonomous of all organization personnel, volunteer or paid. The accountability of the executive

is pervasive. It is not limited to particular persons or clienteles. Since it is organizationally induced, and since organizations are complex internally and in their relationships to the numerous external systems, [chief] administrators are highly exposed to responsibility, and to attributions of responsibility. Whether or not they delegate responsibility, [chief] administrators of organizations are the ones who are ultimately accountable for what is done in and by the organization and its personnel, as well as how and why it is done, and the myriad consequences which follow what is done (Levy, 1979, p. 284).

The position of the chief executive of a social organization is therefore a peculiar one, and often an ambiguous one with implications for the ethics of social work administration of a complex and far-reaching nature.

Since in executives is incorporated the full breadth of ethical responsibility which administrators can carry, I shall be concentrating, in the rest of this book, on the application to executives of the various facets of the ethics of social work administration, emphasizing particularly the administration of voluntary social organizations. Whatever, by way of ethical responsibility, is attributable to the executive of a social organization is attributable at least in part to all other paid organization administrators at all levels of the organizational hierarchy.

The ethical responsibility of administrators of discrete organizational units—like particular departments of a social agency or university, or particular programs in which separate budgets are prepared and accounted for, personnel are independently hired and fired, and even funds are separately raised—corresponds very closely to the ethical responsibility of organization executives. Although the extent and scope of this responsibility, and to a degree its ultimate significance, may be more limited, lower-level administrators have ample opportunity to be unethical—that is, to take advantage of their authority and power in their relationships with others. They have enough opportunity, in fact, to make their positions quite comparable, from an ethical point of view, with that of the chief executive of an organization.

The Executive's Ethical Responsibility

Aside from such ethical responsibility as inheres in the positions of all administrators of a social organization other than the chief executive, whatever ethical responsibility is carried by the chief executive is generally applicable— by formal delegation or by normative ascription or attribution—to all other administrators. They are assumed to act for and in behalf of the chief executive.[1] But executives are ultimately accountable for the omissions and commissions of all administrative personnel. If executives are not invariably punished or censured for the aberrations of subordinates, they are certainly expected to see to it that those subordinates do not commit too many gaffes and to punish and censure them for serious ones, unethical ones included. These options often serve executives well for they provide the means for ridding an organization of superfluous or incompetent or otherwise undesirable or unwelcome staff members.

What this underscores is the relatively greater authority, as well as the relatively greater informal power, with which the executive is invested. But it also underscores the more limited freedom of subordinate administrators. Their freedom, at least, remains within the boundaries of their legitimate authority as overseen by the executive. Still, subordinate administrators, no less than chief executives, are sometimes not above making the most of their illegitimate authority—the authority with which they are invested by *their* subordinates even though they do not have it by organizational definition and administrative assignment.[2]

Caution as well as ethics does require of subordinate administrators, when acting in and on behalf of the employing organization, that they indicate precisely the limits of their authority, and that they avoid actions which might suggest to others that they are acting with greater authority than they actually have. Since the presumption at such junctures is that they are acting for the chief executive, their relationship to the executive becomes the basis for especially sensitive ethical responsibilities and rather imperative principles of ethical conduct.

Chief executives are subject to similar imperatives in relation to the author-

---

[1]"The functions of the executive . . . are those of control, management, supervision, administration in formal organizations ['a *system of consciously coordinated activities or forces of two or more persons'* (Barnard, 1966, p. 73)]. These functions are exercised not merely by high officials in such organizations but by all those who are in positions of control of whatever degree. In the large-scale and complex organizations, the assistants of executives, though not themselves executives, are occupied in the work of these functions" (Barnard, 1966, p. 6).

[2]"There is a strong tendency toward a consensual 'acknowledgment' of the charismatic quality of those in positions of highest authority. So far as authority is visible—this is part of its effectiveness—it does have a self-legitimating consequence. It arouses the attribution of charisma" (Shils, 1965, p. 211).

ity of governing bodies of organizations, and in relation to organization policy and functional boundaries. The issue for both executives and their subordinates is, first, whether actions are authorized under organization policy and purpose at all and, secondly, when those actions are in fact authorized—that is, when they are consistent with policy and purpose—who has the specific authority to carry them out. There are actions that the executive is free to take that subordinates are not, although the executive may be free enough to permit or authorize them to do so. That which the executive is not otherwise authorized or free to do because of the limitations of organization policy or purpose, the executive is ethically as well as administratively obligated to avoid doing pending official action and approval. The executive may of course circumvent formal authority to take advantage of informal opportunities.

Given these constraints and limitations, it is in the organization executive that the ethics of social work administration is prescriptively embodied as a kind of ideal-type, with perhaps variable relevance to other administrative personnel. Not all of the ethical responsibilities of organization executives are necessarily attributable as primary responsibilities to all other administrative personnel, either in degree or in kind, but all other administrative personnel share those responsibilities in some form and in some measure. In addition, they carry particular ethical responsibility in relation to their executive for reasons similar to those which apply to the ethical responsibility of organization personnel to employers and employing organizations, and to colleagues.

The ethical responsibility of executives in relation to their subordinates is of course different in many respects, not only because of differently defined functions and responsibilities, but also because of its very nature and because of its scope and its intensity. A key to one of the major differences is the power implications of the executive's relationship to subordinates. Although other administrators, particularly in large-scale organizations, have access to power as well as authority over *their* subordinates, that is not quite the same thing as ultimate power over all organization personnel:

> A person may be said to have *power* to the extent that he influences the behavior of others in accordance with his own intentions. . . . Most power-holders claim legitimacy for their acts, i.e., they claim the "right to rule" as they do. If the legitimacy of the exercise of power is acknowledged by the subordinated individuals we speak of *legitimate* power; if it is not recognized we call it *coercion* (provided, of course, that the intention of the power-holder is realized). . . . A person whose general position as a power-holder is recognized as legitimate may exercise force, domination, or manipulation . . . the recognition of a powerholder as a legitimate exerciser of power rests on the recognition of the legitimacy of his acts of domination. However, this need not mean that he may not also exercise force or manipulation (Goldhamer and Shils, 1939, pp. 171-173).

There can be little question that, except for an occasional influence which prevents an executive from living up to the potentials of executive authority and power—like being reluctant to use either, and losing both to others all too ready to fill the vacuum—the chief executive, of all staff members of a social organization, has the edge on organizational legitimacy and can use it in unethical as well as ethical ways.[3]

In small organizations, more of the ethical responsibility is lodged in the executive. This is especially true in a one-person administrative operation. The loneliness of executives is therefore not dissipated by the smaller size of an organization or its staff; only the reasons for, and the nature of the isolation changes. In a large-scale voluntary social organization the executive's loneliness is hierarchically ordered. Lacking are horizontal peer relationships in such an organization. The executive is slotted in between board members and subordinates, the more readily to be confronted with ethical issues in relation to both. In a small-scale organization, there are simply few, or even no staff to relate to. The relationship to board members may generate the illusion of intimacy, or the kind of intimacy which can prove problematic in confrontations with ethical issues. The executive's isolation is therefore more qualitatively ordered.

Much of the conflict experienced by executives in confrontations with ethical issues in the larger voluntary social organizations is affected by the volume and nature of their relationships both to board members and to staff members, and the needs and the orientations—both administrative and ideological—which the executives bring to those relationships. But a prime source of the conflict is the ethical expectations for executives, both as they see the expectations and as others see them. Another source of conflict is the values by which executives are guided and influenced in their lives and in their job performance. Still another source is the values which are societally, organizationally, and occupationally associated with administrative responsibility and the responsibility of administrators. These shape and affect the operation of the ethics of social work administration and its impact on executives.

The Power Base of Executive Ethics

The power at the disposal of executives is sometimes more taxing for them emotionally than the vulnerability to which they are actually subject, or to which they perceive themselves to be subject. An interesting difference between executive vulnerability and executive power is that whether merely perceived by executives or actual, their vulnerability is real in its consequences, including its consequences for their ethics. But mere perception of executive

---

[3]"We have learned that danger of tyranny or injustice lurks in unchecked power, not in blended power" (Davis, 1960, p. 54).

power, as contrasted with real or actual power, is effective only if the perception is shared or experienced by those over whom the power may be used. To put this another way, to affect the opportunities or inclination of executives to be unethical, it is enough for executives to perceive themselves to be vulnerable. It is not enough for them to perceive themselves to have certain kinds of power in order to have a similar effect. For that, *others* over whom the power may be wielded have to perceive the executives as having it. But executives do have actual power as well as opportunities to use it, and not infrequently the inclination as well.

Power Based on Responsibility

Executive power, to which the ethics of social work administration would be especially relevant, may be roughly classified under at least three general headings which correspond to the kinds of opportunities that executives have to engage in unethical as well as ethical conduct. The first relates to the responsibility that executives carry for the realization of organization purposes, the execution of organization functions, and the implementation of organization policies. Whatever executives have the assigned responsibility to do in and for their organizations, as employees of those organizations, they, first of all, have the *ethical* duty to do. "The goal of any competent counseling service," for example, "whether it be a family service agency or a mental health center," is "delivery of first-rate clinical services to clients" (Brown, Finkelstein, and Miller, 1979, p. 515). And "the ability of the professional staff to deliver such service depends not only on their skill, maturity, and caring but also on the *tone and character of the agency's administration, beginning with the executive director*" (p. 515; emphasis supplied).

What executives have the duty to do, moreover, gives them the opportunity *not* to do. The failure to do so would constitute unethical conduct since the virtual genesis of ethical responsibility is the duty to perform those functions which one has undertaken to perform.

The basic criterion of judgment affecting the ethics of social organization executives, like the basic criterion of judgment affecting the ethics of any practitioner of any occupation in any organization, is the expectation that that which one is assigned or committed to do in an organization, one will do. The same or similar failure on the part of a person without assigned, assumed, or ascribed responsibility, as compared with a person with such responsibility—although that person may be subject to censure on grounds of general morality—would not subject that person to the sanctions or social disapproval applicable on grounds of occupational ethics to the person with such responsibility.

Like an attorney general who obstructs justice, an ordinary citizen breaks the law in doing so. But the ordinary citizen does not commit the offense to ethics that the attorney general would be chargeable with, since the attorney general is specifically assigned and committed to uphold and implement the law. It is not simply that the attorney general has done something illegal, but that the attorney general has both neglected a duty and prevented its performance. The responsibility to do whatever executives have the responsibility to do, representing also the opportunity not to do it or to do it improperly, is one form of executive power, therefore, which occasions the need for ethics in social work administration.

Power Based on Relationships

Another form of executive power is a function of the executive's relationships to others in an organization. Those relationships—to board members, for example—need not be defined in terms of executive authority, and in fact may involve the authority of others over the executive—authority by which the actions of executives are constrained or limited. Within those relationships, nevertheless, executives can affect others adversely if they so choose. Board members, for example, may rely on executives to attend to matters upon which their own reputations or relationships to others may rest. They may reveal confidences—attitudes towards other board members, for example—which executives can use to discredit them, or to alienate them from other board members. Executives can influence elections and appointments which board members may take quite seriously, and can do so in an underhanded and malicious manner, engaging in what amounts to subversive alignments.

There are others with whom executives of social organizations deal, and whom they can affect in a similarly destructive manner. A high order of ethics is required of executives in those relationships, on one hand to insure attention to responsibility and, on the other, to avoid derelictions of responsibility and abuse of the opportunities and relationships which that responsibility makes possible. The capacity which such responsibility and such relationships create for executives to do or not to do what is called for, or to do it improperly or to the disadvantage of others, though not founded on institutional authority, is a source and locus of executive power.

Power Based on Position

A third source and locus of executive power is the executive's position in the administrative hierarchy of a social organization. This is real, defined, and authorized power over people. Within the organization, at least, and sometimes also beyond the organization when the effects of organization experience of staff members extend to the outermost reaches of their economic and social lives, executives have a lot to say and do about what their subordinates, clients, and others experience, and what they may have the misfortune or opportunity to experience in the future.

To say that executives have access to these types of power, and other types of power as well, is to acknowledge the urgency of ethics in social work administration. Organization members and personnel, community constituents, clients, and others rely on executives to be honest, trustworthy, and fair in dealing with them and with the organization's responsibilities and resources. They expect executives to be honorable in their dealings with them.

All of these things represent reasons for being ethical, and opportunities for being unethical. And in the realm of ethics, as in the realm of administrative practice in general, the prestige with which the status and position of executives cloak them (cf. Barnard, 1946) does not, as Paul Jacobs wrote in an article on the piano music of Debussy, "automatically confer infallibility" (1979, p. 24). It should be no surprise to anyone that it is at least as easy to be fallible about one's ethics as it is to be fallible about the more rationally induced and founded of executive actions, and no doubt much easier.

Personal Values and Ethical Responsibility

Obviously enough, the personal needs, aspirations, insecurities, drives, and so on of executives help to make a difference in the outcome as they contemplate their decisions and actions, and as they cope with their vulnerabilities and their power. Competence—the knowledge, the skill, the ability, and the capacity to make choices and to take actions maximally relevant to organizational purposes and functions, and maximally effective and efficient in implementing those purposes and functions—competence does afford executives access to more of the possible alternatives from which to select those most conducive to the fulfillment of their administrative responsibility. Competence does make judicious choices of action and decisions more likely on the basis of organization purpose and priority, and on the basis of anticipated consequences. But ethics affects, or should affect, the operation of both organization and personal values in the actions and decisions of organization executives.

The ethics of social work administration, by which executives are presumably guided, and upon the basis of which executive actions and decisions may be appraised, along with other more practically oriented bases, amounts to value-oriented prescriptions of executive conduct in the administration of social organizations.

As the social organization's chief administrator, the executive is also the prime carrier of responsibility for the ethics of social work administration in, and on behalf of, the organization. As Chester I. Barnard summarizes a similar point:

> Executive positions a) imply a complex morality, and b) require a high capacity of responsibility, c) under conditions of activity, necessitating

d) commensurate general and specific technical abilities as a *moral* factor . . . in addition there is required e) the faculty of *creating* morals for others (1966, p. 272).

Barnard emphasizes that *"responsibility is the property of an individual by which whatever morality exists in him becomes effective in conduct"* (p. 267) thus underscoring the dimension of individual responsibility for the individual acts and decisions of executives. Social organizations do have attributed to them expectations of an ethical nature, but it is executives who are expected to live up to them, and to see to it that others in the organization live up to them as well.

The burden of these expectations is often almost too much for executives to bear. These expectations are multifarious and multifariously founded. Somewhere in the midst of a confrontation with an issue in ethics, and in contention with value-oriented expectations—that is, the ethics—associated with the issue, impinges the influence of what executives want, or need, or are concerned about, not excluding what they regard as good or necessary for sheer survival or comfort—their own or the organization's, or both. Executives, like other

persons differ not only as to the quality and relative importance of their moral codes or as to their sense of responsibility toward them, or with respect to the effect of incentives, but also because of wide variations in the *number* of codes which govern their conduct. . . . Conflicts of code will increase, as a matter of probability, with increase in number of codes. . . . Conflicts appear to be a product of moral complexity and physical and social activity . . . neither men of weak responsibility nor those of limited capacity can endure or carry the burden of many simultaneous obligations of different types. . . . Conversely, a condition of complex morality, great activity, and high responsibility cannot continue without commensurate ability (Barnard, 1966, pp. 271-272).

Executives and Their Codes

Executives of social organizations, especially the larger and more complex ones but smaller ones as well, are exposed to a multiplicity of organizational, occupational, social, and personal codes, and to a wide range of physical and social activities. Their job generally requires an extensive array of associations and communications—both on and off the job—each with its moral dimensions, each with its implications for administrative ethics. Ability does not guarantee ethics, but ethics is hardly possible—not consistently possible at any rate—without ability: the ability to perceive the value connotations of every responsibility, every association, every relationship, every experience, every organizational issue; and the ability to *choose* to do something ethical about each, and even to *do something* about each.

The Rational Basis of Ethical Judgment

These abilities connote the rational component of ethical judgment and ethical choice. It is not that ethics itself is rational. Ethics, being founded on values—on what is preferred to be done under particular circumstances, in particular relationships, in relation to particular responsibilities, and so on—is, in effect, arbitrary. People and organizations simply *choose* principles of ethical practice, or agree about them, concede them to make sense in and for certain situations. Their application, however, is, or can be—and in the light of executive responsibility, should be—rational. It is as a result of analysis, however rapid, of each situation and its various components, that choice of action, or response, or decision is made. This is something that can be talked about, studied, taught, learned, communicated, explained, evaluated. It is something also that is amenable to guidance.

The actions and decisions of executives of social organizations can thus be rationally contemplated and anticipated, analyzed, and evaluated, and they can be prescribed from the point of view of ethics. The aim in each case will be to discover and propose principles of ethical practice to guide specific administrative actions and decisions, or administrative ethics in general, and to guide the appraisal, the evaluation, and the modification of both. On such processes as these rests the effective genesis of the ethics of social work administration as it may be codified.

Administration: Generic or Specific?

For a concluding consideration for this chapter, I should like to pose what often becomes an inevitable question in discussions of management and administration. As Vincent Vinci phrased it in the title of an article published in *Administrative Management* in 1976, "Can A Good Manager Manage Anything?" (1979-80). Vinci considers this question within the limited framework of industrial management, and yet he expresses doubt about the transferability of managerial and administrative skills from one setting to another, or at least from one set of responsibilities to another. This makes rather ironic, therefore, the frequently articulated plea in recent years that professional managers be hired to administer social service organizations. The implication of this plea seems to be that the peculiar purposes and functions of social organizations notwithstanding, managerial skills have become increasingly and supersedingly urgent for them. That is, the ability to *run* a social organization has begun, in some quarters, to seem more important than the ability to administer and supervise the professional services which the organization has been established to provide for its clients.

"There is an ever-growing need," John J. Stretch asserts, for example, "for increased management skills for human services administrators" (1978, p. 323). "What is conveniently measurable," he goes on to say, "may indeed come to replace what is substantively meaningful." And Harold Lewis makes the following observation:

> Today, as resources contract and demand expands, the call is out for managers . . . managers now enter center stage, as economic distress and political reaction threaten social services in all fields. In the eyes of professionals who must deliver the service, talk of budget cuts, personnel freezes, program retrenchment, and organizational rigidity linked to demands for accountability, is managerial talk. Managers in such trying circumstances find themselves speaking of efficiency, when the professionals—in daily practice—speak of insufficiency (1975, p. 615).

And Paul Abels writes:

> The drastic changes which have taken place in the administration of social welfare programs throughout the country are reflective of a national movement toward centralization and of a movement starting on the Federal level to run programs not on the basis of constituency feedback or client need, but on the basis of centralized control and cost analysis in the guise of scientific management. We see . . . an increasing number of managers trained in systems engineering are administering welfare programs (1973, p. 13).

If it is indeed a problem for executives of social organizations who lack a managerial orientation, to understand principles of management and organization, as Scott Mullis has suggested—and that view is widely shared in the field of social welfare, both public and voluntary—the problem also persists that "professional managers have tremendous difficulty understanding welfare" (1975, p. 31).

In view of all this, as uncertain as the conclusions may be, and given the inconclusive state of available data on the subject, Vinci's response to his own question is especially revealing:

> One reason for the failures [of two managers who were shifted from one sphere of management in which they had done well to another in which they were appraised as having done poorly] and others like them is the rationale used in choosing them. Top management decided primarily on the basis of performance in similar posts. Basically, the people who selected them believed that a successful manager can manage anything (1979-80, p. 26).

Vinci, of course, is reaching for transcendent criteria of managerial competence—criteria which go beyond records of achievement in particular assignments—for a determination of whether individuals are generally "good managers." Nevertheless, his question and his answer are well-taken as far as the issue is concerned of transferability of administrative ability from industrial and political organizations to social organizations. In this respect, it is not only a thorough appreciation of the substance of the social organization's purposes and functions that is required for executive effectiveness and proficiency, but also a profound identification with and investment in the values and ethics which are associated with those purposes and functions. Abels punctuates this consideration and in so doing provides a fitting conclusion for this chapter, even if one is disinclined to accept all of his factual assumptions:

> What is the managerial morality? In fact, the morality lies mainly in giving the organization what it wants; managers are not client advocates. . . .
>
> Management roles are built around getting "things" done, without regard to what these "things" really are. And, as Daniel Katz points out: "Basic changes in (social) system(s) . . . require issue-oriented rather than procedure-oriented managers; i.e., men with genuine knowledge and understanding of the change objectives."
>
> I am not advocating throwing the machines out. We cannot ignore the potential value of good management and a "systems theory" approach to solving human problems. What I am suggesting is that the "human being" must carry more "weight" in the system inputs. The system program must reflect the thinking of the clients and their advocates, rather than the thinking of those who are not really concerned about human needs. . . . Managers of social welfare programs will need to not only be experts in management, but they will have to have a sound orientation in understanding human and social problems as well. . . . We must clarify our ethical and moral framework (1973, p. 15).

It is incumbent upon executives of social organizations to clarify this ethical and moral framework, as well as making it the foundation of their administrative practice. The ethics of social work administration requires of executives of social organizations that they carry out all of their administrative responsibilities within, and with the guidance of this moral and ethical framework, and inspire and encourage others to do likewise.

REFERENCES

Abels, Paul. "The Managers Are Coming! The Managers Are Coming!" *Public Welfare,* 31 (1973), 13-15.

Barnard, Chester I. "Functions and Pathology of Status Systems in Formal Organizations," in William Foote Whyte, ed., *Industry and Society* (New York: McGraw Hill, 1946), 46-83.

Barnard, Chester I. *The Functions of the Executive* (Cambridge, Mass,: Harvard University Press, 1966).

Brown, Helen Sauer, Finkelstein, Non D., and Miller, Walter D. "An Innovative Approach to Selecting An Executive Director," *Social Casework,* 60 (1979), 515-519.

Davis, Kenneth Culp. *Administrative Law and Government* (St. Paul, Minn.: West Publishing, 1960).

Goldhamer, Herbert, and Shils, Edward A. "Types of Power and Status," *The American Journal of Sociology,* 45 (1939), 171-182.

Jacobs, Paul. "On Playing the Piano Music of Debussy," *Keynote* (WNCN), September, 1979, pp. 18-22, 24.

Levy, Charles S. "The Ethics of Management," *Administration in Social Work,* 3 (1979), 277-288.

Lewis, Harold. "Management in the Nonprofit Social Service Organization," *Child Welfare,* 54 (1975), 615-623.

Mullis, Scott. "Management Applications to the Welfare System," *Public Welfare,* 33 (1975), 31-34.

Shils, Edward A. "Charisma, Order, and Status," *American Sociological Review,* 30 (1965), 199-213.

Stretch, John J. "Increasing Accountability for Human Services Administrators," *Social Casework,* 59 (1978), 323-329.

Vinci, Vincent. "Can a Good Manager Manage Anything?" *Readings in Management 79/80 Annual Editions* (Service Dock, Guilford, Ct.: Dushkin Publishing Group), 26-27. Reprint from *Administrative Management,* September, 1976.

VI. THE EXECUTIVE AND THE ORGANIZATION

In a review of research on organizational leadership, Burton Gummer alludes to the major role which is played by executives of organizations in determining the overall effectiveness of the organizations (1979, p. 359). The social organization may not be the "elongated shadow" of the executive, as Gummer suggests, but, from a functional and operational point of view, the executive is certainly at least a truncated or symbolic reflection of what the organization is and does and how it does what it does.

The Social Organization Executive as Organization Symbol

This is the empirical view of the status and role of the social organization executive when it can be factually verified on the basis of observation. That is, this is how an executive may look to an objective observer when the executive is observed to function in a manner which coincides with what is expected of a social organization by way of manifest purpose, structure, operation, practices, and procedures. Prescriptively, on the other hand, the executive is supposed—and therefore expected—to reflect in conduct and practice that which is expected of the organization according to its avowed and assumed purposes and functions. In effect, therefore, the executive of a social organization is accountable—it is the executive's ethical responsibility—for whatever may be attributed to the organization as institutional responsibility.

The executive is ethically responsible for making possible if not likely the realization of the organization's purposes in a manner maximally considerate of its resources, and maximally sensitive to the impact of all procedures and practices on persons in the organization and affected by it. The executive is responsible for getting the organization's work done, or seeing to, and facilitating, its doing. The executive is also responsible for doing so in a manner which is responsive to the values by which the organization and its purposes and functions are assumed to be guided—both as an administrator who is in the employ of the organization, and as an affiliate of the particular profession or occupation with which the executive may be identified. With reference to the latter, what this emphasizes is that the executive who is a social worker, for example, is accountable for such ethics as may be attributed to administrators of social organizations in general, but also the ethics attributable to social workers as social workers. Although this cannot as readily be said to apply to the social worker who happens to manage an industrial enterprise like an automobile producing and selling corporation, it does apply to the social worker who manages a social organization, primarily because of the greater congruence between the social purposes of the social organization and the social purposes of the social work profession. It would also be applicable to the executive of a social work program in an industrial organization.

The Normative Foundation of Administrative Ethics

This is not to suggest that executives of industrial organizations are not bound by principles of ethical administrative practice, whether formalized by a code of ethics or not; only that the principles are differently founded and reflect some differences in substance and form because of differences in purposes and functions as between industrial and social organizations. The following commentary by former Secretary of the Treasury W. Michael Blumenthal makes this quite evident:

> The rash of disclosures of corporate bribes and other illegal payments here and abroad has provoked a chorus of questions about ethics, morality, and the modern corporate executive. In fact, our entire economic system is being scrutinized as never before . . . neither more government control of business nor the breakup of big corporations will lead automatically to a higher standard of morality in business . . . the changes that have taken place in the business environment can be divided into two broad categories: The first involves the new expectations that society has imposed on industry. The second concerns the complexity of the problems confronting executives today.
>
> The result is that the decision-making process in business has become far more complicated than it used to be . . . many of yesterday's executive prerogatives have been circumscribed by these changes. . . . Society has imposed minimum standards of conduct that all businesses must meet as a condition of operating in the first place (1979-80, pp. 270-271).

Although perhaps for different reasons, and on different grounds, the prerogatives of executives of social organizations have been, and continue to be, circumscribed. Their decision-making—particularly with respect to issues in ethics that arise in their daily administrative practice—is hardly less complicated than that of their corporate counterparts. The essential reason is not simply that society is watching them more closely. It is rather that, because they run social organizations, they tend to be more subject to general scrutiny, and tend to be held to stricter expectations than are corporate executives.

The Codification of Ethics for Business and Social Organizations

As I have already suggested, moreover, more of the expectations of an ethical nature which are attributed to business executives derive from the moral norms of society—not a few of which contradict one another—and more of the expectations of an ethical nature which are attributed to executives of social organizations derive from occupational and social service norms.

The distinction between the two is not all that sharp, however. Business executives also classify themselves, or are classified by others occupationally, as managers or administrators to whom principles of ethical practice are applicable, and for whom principles of ethical practice have been and continue to be codified. And business organizations have developed, and continue to develop, codes of ethics of variable form and substance, and in variable stages of refinement, each of which provides a moral framework for the conduct of executives in those organizations. There has been some movement toward collaborative efforts among business and industrial organizations to fashion interorganizational codes of ethics, but little stock is evidently put "in codes other than the ones companies formulate for themselves," so that such efforts have not only met with little or no success, but have also been questioned (cf. *Business Week,* 1976).

Whether the efforts at codification have been successful or not, or independent or not, and whether or not they have been a response to public and governmental reaction to recent incidents of bribery, skulduggery, and venality on the part of business and industry on the national and international scene, expectations of an ethical nature are applied to business organizations and their executives. In addition, of course, associations of business people such as jewelers, advertisers, marine tradespersons, forwarders and receivers, building custodians, and others have compiled principles of ethical practice relevant to executive functioning in their enterprises.

The "Business" Ethics of Social Organization "Business"

As far as business operations are concerned, the executive function in social organizations may be properly subsumed under the category of the executive function in all organizations, including business and industrial organizations, at least as far as its ethics is concerned. Whatever is expected of, or prescribed for executives in business and industrial organizations, according to existing codes and custom and usage, therefore, may be assumed to be applicable to executives of social organizations.

Perhaps it is more accurate to say that what is generic about administrative ethics applies both to social organizations and to business and industrial organizations. But the obverse of this proposition may not as readily be assumed: What is applicable to the executive function in social organizations is not in all respects applicable to the executive function in business and industrial organizations. The differences in purposes and functions of social organizations, as compared with business and industrial organizations, require differences in their ethics, although both are bound by some ethics in common. The business and managerial practices and procedures required of social organizations, however, are in fundamental respects comparable with those in business and industrial organizations. As far as ethics is concerned, therefore, similar expectations apply, to the extent that social organizations are engaged in practices comparable to those of business and industrial organizations.

To put this more boldly, whatever by way of ethical conduct is expected of executives in business and industry is also expected of executives of social organizations, but not everything that is expected of executives of social organizations is expected of executives of business and industrial organizations. It is not only that principles of ethical practice are not similarly applicable or relevant to each of these settings. It is also that expectations differ. In this connection I should also emphasize the distinction between expectations which are simply normative, and expectations which are occupationally imperative and, at their most effective in relation to the social purpose which they are designed to serve, enforceable.

The differences between expectations ascribed to social organization executives and those ascribed to executives of business and industrial organizations, are graphically summarized by Harold Lewis:

> It is important to clarify the situation of social service administrators; what it is we want help with, and what factors in our circumstances condition the use we can make of help that may be provided. We come from a culture very different from that of the business manager. We operate nonprofit organizations and can, with little effort, spend for good purposes more than we have, thereby incurring a deficit, but no loss in profit. When our consumers no longer need our services, an optimistic interpretation is that success has been achieved; this is hardly the case in business when customers stop buying a firm's product. In the social service organization concern for fairness often takes precedence over efficiency. The service ethic considers unequal advantage justified only if it raises the expectations of the least advantaged. Since the most disadvantaged are also more likely to experience difficulty in making appropriate use of opportunities, special and costly effort may be required to reach out to them. This, despite the fact that other claimants who do not need this special effort are sufficient in number to absorb totally the available resources. What business would spend resources to attract the most difficult to serve and usually most deprived customer when there are more than enough cooperative and affluent customers prepared to buy all it has to sell?
>
> In business, when competition doesn't bring efficiency, adversity will. In social service, rarely does competition compel efficiency, and adversity is not likely to be the result of a client taking his business elsewhere. Given our lack of resources, selective inefficiency may be a necessity for organizational survival (1975, pp. 615-616).

An item which appeared in *Business Week* a few years ago suggests the operation of some of these differences, from the business point of view, even as it emphasizes the growing attention to, and concern about, the morality of business and industry:

> Policy statements on business ethics pour forth from corporations in the wake of almost daily disclosures that some of this country's most distinguished executives were themselves "overly ambitious employees" who did not care how results were obtained, even if it meant breaking the law . . . there are welcome signs of tighter controls, of belated efforts to establish a higher moral tone throughout management and, in a few companies, of a serious grappling with questions of right and wrong that go beyond the simple strictures of bribing politicians. . . . Pressure is also building, from inside business and out, for a national or international code of business ethics. . . . Most executives, however, put little stock in codes other than the ones companies formulate for themselves. . . . One problem is that any general code would have to be so watered down to gain general acceptance that it would be all but useless. . . . In the final analysis, codes of good conduct—and enforcement of those codes—will be up to individual companies. . . .
>
> What business must understand today is that the public has a right to demand much more. When executives at the summit of some of the nation's most prestigious and powerful companies fail such an elementary moral test [e.g., illegal bribery], shareholders, workers, and customers can legitimately wonder what else is going on in the executive suite (1976).

The Moral Obligations of Social Organizations and Their Executives

When it comes to the morality of the social organization's executive suite, the public and others do more than wonder for, as service organizations, they are subject to considerable extra-legal scrutiny and held to greater extra-legal expectations. And so are their executives.

To review the expectations for social organizations, and the consequent ethical responsibility of their executives,[1] the following questions may be posed:

1. In the light of existing needs and accessible as well as available resources, do the purposes of the social organization merit the organiza-

---

[1]Although the social organization is more than the group of managers that Peter Drucker says it is, one can certainly agree with him when he says that "The institution itself is, in effect, a fiction" (1977, p. 11). The social organization, like any organization, is what the people in it make of it, and do in it or on its behalf.

tion's attention and the expenditure of the personal, professional, and material resources which are invested in those purposes?

2. Does the social organization consistently, effectively, and efficiently address the purposes for which it has been created and for which it continues to be maintained? Are those purposes still valid?

3. Do the functions which are performed in the social organization conduce to the achievement of its avowed and socially sanctioned purposes?

4. Do the structure of the social organization, its policies, its procedures, its practices, and the recruitment, deployment, and supervision of its personnel, and others of its approaches and activities, conduce to the effective, economical, and ethical implementation of its functions?

5. Are the policies, procedures, operations, and practices of the social organization responsive to, and reflective of, the values by which its services and its social functions are presumed to be guided?

6. Are the relationships among the staff members of the social organization, and between them and the organization's executives, as well as those between its board and staff members, guided by the values and ethics by which its services to its clientele and membership are guided?

In these questions are contained the clues to the ethics which may be prescribed as a matter of occupational responsibility for the executive of a social organization in relation to the organization as a whole. Despite the degree of congruence that occurs between the ethics that may be prescribed for business executives and the ethics which may be prescribed for social organization executives, these questions connote different or additional criteria for the evaluation of the ethics of social organization executives, primarily because of the relative emphasis which is placed on the social responsibility of social organizations and their executives. (Compare, however, Silk and Vogel, 1976; Nelson and Campbell, 1972; and Abouzeid and Weaver, 1979/80.) That which is imperative for the social organization and its executive is rather incidental for business executives. For the social organization and its executive, social responsibility is the main job, as it were. Effective and relevant service to the clientele of a social service organization is a function of that responsibility. For the business and industrial organization and its executive, profit, productivity, and measurable outcomes are its main job. Social responsibility, in effect, represents the social constraints and influences in doing it.

Social organizations can well use the "great man" version of leadership in their executives that is so widely valued in business and industry, since, as I have suggested, many of their operations are business operations—very practical, technical operations. But in social organizations these are designed primarily to make service possible as well as effective. For business and industry, the business of business, as it has been said, is primarily business. Executive success in business and industry is therefore differently measured and valued than it is in social organizations, although a growing preoccupation in social organizations with economic proficiency, fiscal productivity, and technical efficiency presages a tempering of this difference. What begin as means to service ends often become ends in themselves. But this appears to be more a happenstance of experience and reality than a consequence of philosophy.

So if Leon Reinharth can ask—and properly—"Can an executive who succeeds in one organization transfer that success automatically to any other firm?" (1979/80, p. 32), one can justly ask whether an executive competent in business and industry is automatically competent to administer a social organization. One should certainly ask whether the ethics of the executive in business and industry is sufficient for the purposes of social organizations. The "great man" theory of leadership, according to Reinharth, "describes a business or industrial manager who has the ability to be an effective leader under a variety of situations." But he concludes that "only a small percentage of managers can be classified as 'great man' leaders." If that is the case, one must doubt that the crossing from business or industry to the social organization is any more surefooted, especially when the consideration is not merely administrative competence but administrative ethics.

But I do not mean this to be an empirical judgment. Rather, my intention is to stress the necessity of an orientation peculiar to administrative ethics in social organizations, and the need for especially designed and acquired personal equipment for the purpose. In this connection, Reinharth, in effect, makes an *a fortiori* case for the differences in requirements for administrative ethics in social organizations as compared with administrative ethics in business and industrial organization, for he says—within the exclusive framework of the latter—"Our task is therefore to isolate one set of key leadership elements required for successful performance in one type of organization and another set for another kind of organization." The assumption in relation to administrative ethics is not that one is better or worse than the other; only that they are different in significant ways.

Morality is hardly the exclusive province of social organization executives. Herbert A. Simon and his colleagues were not discussing executives of social organizations but what they said applies to them, when they wrote:

> No knowledge of administrative techniques . . . can relieve the administrator from the task of moral choice—choice as to organization goals and methods and choice as to his treatment of the other human beings in his organization. His code of ethics is as significant a part of his equipment as an administrator as is his knowledge of administrative behavior, and no amount of study of the "science" of administration will provide him with this code. . . . Premises that underlie any administrative choice . . . involve two distinct kinds of elements: *value elements* and *factual elements* (1958, pp. 24, 58).

Executive Loyalty and Devotion to the Social Organization

Not unlike executives of business and industrial organizations, executives of social organizations, first and foremost, owe to the organizations the same kind of loyalty and devotion that any practitioner owes to any client, and any employee owes to an employer. For the purposes of ethics, these relationships resemble one another, as do the ethical responsibilities which derive from them. The loyalty and devotion owed by the social organization executive to the organization may be placed at the primary level of ethical responsibility in any hierarchical ordering of administrative ethics—leaving aside for the moment any contravening considerations. A necessary starting point in the analysis of any issue in administrative ethics, as in occupational ethics in general, is the identification of primary responsibility, with the customary proviso, "other things being equal," which they of course rarely are. Such loyalty and devotion do not inevitably and invariably signify "my organization right or wrong," but they do connote a high order of priority—high enough to require compelling considerations before neglect of them or deviation from them can be justified.

This is not a simple demand because of the extreme complexity of executive responsibility in social organizations. The executive of a social organization is never exempt from the ethical responsibility to be loyal and devoted to the organization, and to serve it—as it is put in the code of ethics of the National Association of Social Workers—with "determination, and the maximum application of professional skill and competence" (1979). The most that can be said, with any justification, of a deviation from this moral expectation, should the executive fail to honor it and live by it in any particular respect, is that another responsibility or another value superseded it—the responsibility to a social service client, for example, when the executive is also a social worker by profession. A case would then have to be made—should a complaint be lodged against the executive, for example—in justification of the deviation. Ideally, of course, the justification should precede the wayward (for so it must be regarded) action rather than follow it.

The process of ethical decision-making, before the fact, includes the consideration, the weighing, and the *weighting* of all conceivable factors relevant and applicable to executive action and intervention in administrative practice situations. The first line of attack for the executive—when a practice situation calls for a carefully considered choice of action or intervention—is to consider ways in which the executive's professional and administrative responsibility can be most effectively and efficiently carried out and yet done so in a manner most consistent with the principle of maximum loyalty, devotion, determination, and the maximum application of administrative skill and competence. The question to be addressed, in other words, is: How can the executive be most responsive to this ethical responsibility, and yet do the required administrative job most ethically, skillfully, and competently? The second line of attack is occasioned by the need, as perceived by the executive, to put relatively less emphasis on loyalty and devotion to the organization, if not to neglect it altogether, because something else—another interest or another value like service to organization clients—is regarded as more important or more urgent. This need does arise in administrative practice; nor does the alternative of deviating from the principle of loyalty and devotion always represent a betrayal of the organization, although it may very well be just that. In that case, deviation from the principle may not constitute a simple preference but an absolute imperative. The reasons have to be compelling, for the choice of the executive is that between being "for" the organization and "against" it.

Sometimes, however, the choice of the executive is one among alternatives, all of which are consistent with the executive's ethical responsibility in and to the organization. This may, in part, be a consequence of the organization's multiple and sometimes conflicting objectives, some related to its declared social purposes and functions, but others related more to such ends, for example, as its own survival. The executive is responsible for both, but both cannot always be gracefully or ethically accommodated.

An illustration of the effect of such a conflict is the formulation in a social organization of policies and procedures which suit the convenience of its leadership, and effect economies which are not entirely imperative in the light of other available options. At the same time, these policies and procedures sometimes have—as the executive sees the situation—the unfortunate consequence of reducing access to the organization's social services for those among its clientele who are most in need of them. The executive, having occupational as well as ethical responsibility in relation to both, is not always strategically in a position to validate a preference for either.

Warner and Havens characterize the problem for the executive in terms of organizational inclination which is expressed through its policies and procedures to which the executive is assumed to be committed:

> One of the central problems in organizational analysis is to account for the tendency for some organizations to concentrate upon activities and programs that contribute relatively little to the attainment of their major goals. The most common form of this tendency is goal displacement, in which the major goals claimed by the organization are neglected in favor of goals associated with building or maintaining the organization (1968, p. 539).

The executive, in such a case, is, as a matter of ethical responsibility, supposed to adhere to organization policy and procedures (cf. NASW, 1979, item IV L). But the executive, also as a matter of ethical responsibility, is supposed to advance and facilitate the implementation of the organization's service purposes. Either choice is ethically "correct," but if both cannot be accommodated simultaneously, one must be preferred. It is then incumbent upon the executive to consider in advance, and be able to demonstrate after the fact, that the choice ultimately made merited the priority accorded to it.

This is hardly the end of the line, however, for it is equally incumbent upon the executive to make such provisions, and to engage in such efforts, as will make possible the increasing convergence of organization policies and procedures, on one hand, and organization purposes and functions, on the other. These incumbencies are both immediate and long-range ones. The immediate one is to attempt to increase accessibility to service while staying within the boundaries of organization policy and procedures. The long-range one is to channel efforts for change in the direction of revised policies and procedures increasingly congruent with the organization's service purposes and functions. Both are as much a function of the executive's art and skill as an administrator, as a function of the executive's ethics.

The Organization and the Community

An illustration may be offered of what may be described as an ethical conflict of the internal-external variety for the executive of a social organization. Expected of the executive, according to the principle of loyalty and devotion to the organization, is attention to whatever of an administrative nature may be required for the maintenance and survival of the organization, and for the sustenance of its continued health and well-being as an organization. Also expected of the executive is attention to the collective needs and requirements of the community in which the social organization is located, to which the organization is also assumed to be committed as a social organization. The executive is likely to face a conflict of ethical responsibility if the local community organization—a federation, say, or a united fund—of which the social organization is a constituent member finds—let us assume on valid grounds—that the organization is duplicating already and adequately available services. Or if the community organization finds that services which it offers can more readily, more economically, more effectively, more efficiently, and more conveniently be provided to clientele in need of them by merging the social organization with another or, perhaps, by having it absorbed by another. (This, of course, makes somewhat tenuous the assumption that the grounds for merger or other extreme action are valid, for such actions are not always so benevolently motivated. However, the assumption is reasonable for the purposes of the illustration.)

The executive who represents the social organization is ethically pressed to represent the best interests of the organization. As employer, the organization *relies* on the executive to represent its best interests, however they are seen by the organization, and *trusts* the executive to represent them. At the same time, the executive, as a leader of a social organization, is obliged—it is also an ethical responsibility—to conserve the community's resources, and to increase and improve services to community constituents. As Harold Stein posed the problem for the executive in his casebook in public administration (1952), although the social organization is viewed in the community as institutionally committed to these goals, it is the executive who incurs the ethical responsibility to cooperate in the attempts to achieve them. In the case of the voluntary social organization, board members may be expected to err on the side of institutional loyalty. Although, in effect, trustees of the community, their vested interest in their organization is more likely to be tolerated. Other board members, including board members of the community organization, many of whom also double as board members of other social organizations, are more likely to be sympathetic toward them than they might be inclined to be toward the organization executive. This is more certainly the case when the organization's board members are also among the community's major contributors and prestigious leaders. (If they are "major" enough, in fact, the issue may not even arise, providing, of course, they have a vested interest in the organization's survival.) As far as the executive is concerned, however, it is a different story. The executive is more likely to be held to account both for the survival of the organization *and* the support of the community's collective interests. In Stein's rather dramatic terms:

> Administrator, agency, program—all are subject to attack . . . Politics [and politics operates no less in voluntary organizations than in governmental organizations. C.S.L.] involves ethics and benefits and power; it is the resolution of the contending forces in society. In this light we see the administrator as an agent of society making choices that affect the well-being of society. . . . The administrator must rely on his own system of values—his feeling for what is right—his judgment of what to emphasize, or what to play down—his sense of justice and fair play. The fundamental safeguard against an administrator's arbitrary and unethical conduct is the fact that public administration [like the administration of any social organization. C.S.L.], especially in a democracy, circumscribes the range of values which the administrator can observe. For the making of value judgments by the administrator is part and parcel of the whole system. Every act of political response that can be weighed, in terms of its significance for survival, has value connotations as well (1952, pp. xvi-xvii).

In social organizations it is not only the executive's personal and private values that count. In fact, those values may contradict the values by which the executive may be expected to be guided as a matter of occupational responsibility. The question for the executive will be whether the guidance necessary for ethical choice will come from ethical responsibility to the organization, which derives preferentially from a definition of administrative responsibility to the organization; or from ethical responsibility to the society, which derives from an assumption of responsibility to the society, as reflected in the interests of current and prospective clientele. It is particularly the latter responsibility to which the planning function of community organizations is addressed:

> Service capability considerations . . . must play a significant role in determining the nature and basis of organizational relationships . . . Interorganizational cooperation clearly serves to enhance service delivery [which may be more a prescriptive than an empirical observation, C.S.L.]. However, such capability exchange is not always possible and conflict over organizational domain often politicizes interorganizational relationships in the human services. . . . The focus of interorganizational planning needs to be centered upon *the effect on service effectiveness generated by interorganizational relationships.* Like the clinician, the manager must develop a professional commitment to ensure the highest quality of service. . . . It is this commitment that makes management in the human services different from management in other organizational contexts (Miringoff, 1980, pp. 165-166, 175, 194).

Although some organizational objectives reflect a responsiveness to institutional responsibility to society and to present and prospective clienteles, this responsibility, as vocationally assigned or ascribed to the executive, is not customarily accorded higher priority than that to the organization. On the contrary, since the executive works for, and is employed by the organization, the most plausible assumption that can be made is that the executive owes highest priority to responsibility to the organization. Such obligations as the executive may have to the society as a whole derive primarily from the executive's occupational status rather than the executive's position in the organization.

The NASW Code of Ethics, for example, includes a section on "The Social Worker's Ethical Responsibility to Society," followed by the specification: "Promoting the General Welfare—The social worker should promote the general welfare of society" (1979). The social worker who is the executive of a social organization is therefore expected to weigh the interests of society and its constituents along with the interests of the organization. The interests of the organization, however, would appear to merit relatively greater immediate concern since the relationship of the executive to the organization is specifically and institutionally defined—this notwithstanding the organization's own responsibility to society as it may be reflected in the organization's objectives and for which the executive incurs administrative responsibility. The obligation of the executive to society is a rather generalized and diffuse expectation attributed to the executive primarily as a member of the social work profession—hardly as enforceable as the obligation to the organization which is contractual, whether written into an employment contract or not.

Similar considerations would affect the role of any other executive who is affiliated with any other occupational group the code of ethics, or the customs and usage of which, included a similar provision. Enforceable or not, such a principle of ethical practice would at the very least represent a valued guide or inspiration to the executive's conduct in office if not an influence on it. As Simon and his colleagues put it within the context of public administration:

> A professional code [of ethics] limits the ends or goals to which the skills of the profession may be applied. Thus it frequently happens that professional codes come into conflict with the organizational goals and values. When this happens, hierarchical and even legislative controls may be quite impotent (1958, p. 546).

The executive's "professional code" might very well require—as the codes of ethics of most human service professions do—an investment of effort and support for the collectivity of a community or of a group of cooperating agencies. Such a collectivity might well conclude, with considerable substantiation, that the executive's organization ought to merge with another organization and perhaps even be absorbed by it, in order to conserve resources and perhaps improve services. But the executive's code would no doubt also require of the executive vigorous effort and support for the executive's organization in its own self-interest.

Suppose, for example, that the executive officially represents the organization in the community organization of which the organization is a constituent member—a federation, for example, or a community council. The executive has ethical responsibility to the organization as its representative, and to the community organization as a cooperating participant. Both represent moral obligations, but since the executive is an employee of the organization and is relied on to represent the organization's interest loyally and competently, the obligation to it is a relatively greater one. From an ethical point of view, therefore, the executive owes the employing organization a degree of priority.

This does not preclude efforts to change the organization's perspective in relation to the needs and circumstances of the community as a whole, if not to change the perspective of the community organization in line with the self-interest of the executive's organization by producing a proposition which accommodates that self-interest while accomplishing the service ends in view. One mistake that the executive must scrupulously avoid is acting on a misguided notion of ethical conduct by assuming a role more appropriate for the executive of the community organization. To paraphrase the punchline of a

favorite anecdote of Adlai Stevenson's, if the community organization executive is attentive to the ethical responsibility due the community organization,
and if the organization executive is attentive to the ethical responsibility due the
community organization, who will be attending to the ethical responsibility due
the executive's employing organization? Both within the social organization,
and in the relationships of the organization to other organizations and to the
community as a whole, the executive, in Peter Drucker's words, "has to manage and improve what already exists and is already known" (1977, p. 32).
Drucker is especially interested in business management and in the relationship
of the administrator to, and practice in, the organization. However, the principle he enunciates is equally applicable to the executive of the social organization,[2] with the added consideration that the executive of the social organization
has ethical responsibility for the well-being of those in need of service in the
entire community, and not only those served by the organization. The executive
also has ethical responsibility for the effects of what the organization does or
does not do, and how the organization does or does not do it.

What Drucker adds, as "another dimension" of the managerial task in the
organization, seems especially suited to the administrative task of the social
organization executive for he says, "The *administrative* job of the manager is to
optimize the yield from [existing] . . . resources." In view of the executive's
social function in a social organization which, given its social purposes (services and programs), includes a measure of social responsibility, the resources
about which the executive owes concern, and in relation to which the executive
owes ethical responsibility, are not only those of the organization but those
generally available and accessible for the purposes the organization seeks to
serve, and the functions the organization undertakes to perform.

Social responsibility—both the social organization's and the executive's—
would signify a concern that these purposes and functions be well and efficiently addressed, however and by whomsoever that can best be done. Again,
this may not be the way things are, but ethics suggests how they might and
ought to be, and executives of social organizations are often in a strategic
position to help make them so. To apply Drucker's neat epigram to the question

---

[2]"Management is the specific organ of the new institution, whether business enterprise, or
university, hospital or armed service, research lab or government agency. If institutions are to
function, managements must perform . . . all these institutions have in common the management
function, the management task, and the management work. In all of these there is a group of people
whose function it is to 'manage,' and who have legal power and responsibility as managers. In all
of them there is the same task: making the institution perform. And in all of them this requires
doing specific work; setting objectives, goals and priorities; organizing; staffing; measuring results;·
communicating and decision making, and so on. . . .

The non-business, public-service institutions do not need management less than business. They
may need it more" (Drucker, 1977, pp. 10-12).

of the executive's own effectiveness and efficiency, "Efficiency is concerned with doing things right. Effectiveness is doing the right things."

Richard M. Titmuss summarizes these issues quite pointedly:

> The problems involved in the study of Social Administration [which is "concerned with the study of certain human organizations and formal structures (and choices between them) which deliver or provide what we call 'social services' . . . the methods by which available resources (in cash and in kind) are brought to bear on socially recognized needs"] are not wholly problems of method. There is a value component in discussions about selectivity and universality—a subject (if it is a subject) which cannot be debated at all without considering both aims and methods (1974, p. 50).

The Executive's Conflicts of Ethical Choice

The situations I have described are likely to generate tensions for the executive of the social organization, tensions reminiscent of Launcelot Gobbo's state of mind in *The Merchant of Venice* when he finds himself poised on the abyss between loyalty to his master and loyalty to his Christian confreres. Such tensions usually arise out of the necessity to choose not so much between a "right" and a "wrong" course of action, as between two "right"—or ethical—courses of action. They emanate from conflicts of loyalties, not only loyalty to the employing organization and loyalty to community, but a whole array of loyalties—to clients and prospective clients; to contributors of funds and public and private institutions which grant funds; to whatever professional or occupational group the executive is identified with; and so on.

Cues for the alleviation of the tensions experienced by executives in administrative situations which require decisions or actions, and which carry ethical connotations, do not in practice always come from behavioral expectations or principles of ethical conduct more formally codified by organizations and occupational groups, including associations of administrators. Such sources do afford guidance for executives, and perhaps even inspiration, but it is ultimately they who must exercise such discretion as they have the authority, the responsibility, and the freedom to exercise in applying the principles of ethical practice thus made available to them.

These principles also become available for use in evaluating the conduct of executives, and at times in disciplining them if they are found to offend any of these principles—providing reasonable discrimination can be made between that which is competent in administrative practice, and that which is ethical, for there are times when it cannot be both.

When laws exist which govern the conduct of executives—like the Foreign Corrupt Practices Act of 1977, for example, and laws governing the conduct of public agency executives—then the laws may be applied as well.[3] But a primary purpose of ethics, whether codified or not, is to influence or constrain the conduct of practitioners and, depending on the enforceability of prescribed principles of ethical practice, to compel ethical conduct even when no law exists to do so. Contrariwise, when the law does exist which permits or encourages unethical conduct, the issue for the practitioner to resolve is whether to transgress the law in order to be ethical.

An illustration would be a legal requirement that a social worker, in court testimony, reveal the confidences of a client, an act proscribed by the NASW Code of Ethics. A social worker may choose to go to jail for contempt of court rather than betray the client.

Prescribed and codified principles of ethical administrative practice are unfortunately not the only, nor always the most compelling influence on the ethics of social organization executives or of social organizations in general:

> There are certain types of value premises that we will encounter repeatedly in organization decisions. Perhaps the most important of these are 1) the organization objectives, 2) the criterion of efficiency, 3) standards of fair play, and 4) the personal values of the individual making the decision. . . . The choice an individual will make in any situation is compounded from 1) his skills, knowledge, character, and personality . . . and 2) the specific influences that act upon him at the time of decision (Simon, Smithburg, and Thompson, 1958, pp. 59, 66).

---

[3]The conflict between the loyalty to employing organizations which is expected of organization executives, and the social responsibility which is expected particularly of social organization executives, is suggested by the second look taken at the Foreign Corrupt Practices Act by the Carter administration when the Act appeared to be having an effect on overseas business. The law made it a crime for American corporations to bribe foreign officials in order to obtain business. It also prohibited falsification of accounting records to obscure bribes. The White House's Export Disincentives Task Force became concerned about the loss of trade as a result. Its recommendations to then-President Carter "call for immediate weakening and eventual abandonment of key provisions in the law that prohibits payment of bribes overseas by American corporations" (*The New York Times,* June 12, 1979). The reason, ostensibly, that the law was passed was that overseas bribery—any bribery—constitutes an offense to public policy, and public policy is supposed to represent the values by which public actions are presumably to be guided. It is the mirror image of social responsibility. Ethics—in business or out—is nothing if it is not sacrifice. It is either giving up something in order to do what is morally "right," or avoiding an unfair advantage in order not to do something that is morally "wrong." Sometimes it even means losing some business or making less profit. Normatively speaking, despite the relatively high priority business executives are expected to assign to loyalty to the organization, they are still expected to consider their broader social responsibility. The only difficulty is that sometimes this gives way to expediency, which it may also do in social organizations.

The Influence of Personal Values on Administrative Decisions

Many types of values influence the decisions of social organization executives. Personal values are especially influential, but they are not always reliable, not from the point of view of ethics, unless they happen to coincide in appreciable measure with the values prescribed as premises for ethical practice in the administration of social organizations (cf. Levy, 1976). To cite A. L. Rowse's reading of Flannery O'Connor, "it is at moments of emergency, of extreme tension that people reveal their true character" (1978, Vol. III, p. 8). And the true character of executives, like the true character of other practitioners, is not always in harmony with their ethical responsibility. The good intentions of social organization executives notwithstanding, their decisions in confrontations with ethical issues require a kind of self-transcendance into the higher reaches of ethical responsibility.

> Decisions may be made not only with greater or less skill but also with or without "responsibility"; and though we often differ in our judgments of how skillfully another has reached a decision, we are quick to sense and seldom dispute whether he has made it "responsibly" or not . . . judgment and decision, though mental activities of individuals, are also part of a social process (Vickers, 1965, pp. 14-15).

The ethics of social work administration is clearly a social process in which social responsibility is implicated. The decisions of executives of social organizations, when issues in ethics are confronted, cannot validly be based only on what executives think is "right." They require substantiation on other, less subjective grounds, including the purposes and functions of the organizations, and the executives' role and responsibility in them. They include as well the stakes and interests of others who may be affected and to whom executives owe ethical responsibility.

What Felice Perlmutter seems to be describing as an empirically authenticated fate of social organizations may be more accurately regarded—at least as a generalization—as a prescription for organizational development, and a framework for the fulfillment of the ethical responsibility of social organization executives. It may or may not be generally and inevitably true that social organizations proceed chronologically or developmentally through the three developmental stages of institutional life that Perlmutter conceptualizes— namely, self-interest, professionalism, and social interest (1969)—but it is certainly a matter of ethical responsibility for executives of such organizations to encourage, inspire, and help them attain the stage at which they focus increasingly on their social responsibility and decreasingly on their self-interest.

The clarity of the value framework is the basic ingredient which informs the organizational structure [of a social organization] and its attendant processes. . . . The first stage of self-interest focuses on the development of a distinctive organizational identity and crystallization of basic commitments . . . and addresses itself to the unsolved social problem in its environment. An ideology is made explicit as the initial formalization process occurs. . . . The specification of institutional mission links the social problem and the ideology with the particular system's identity, as its goals and policies are defined. . . .

The shift to the second stage results from new external conditions that affect the developmental character of the agency. . . . Given the value framework of the first stage, the agency seeks to develop its techniques and to obtain relevant information to increase its resources in order to better perform its central tasks; this results in a focus on means rather than ends. The investment in professionalism is ultimately realized as new relationships develop between the agency and other professional organizations in the broader system. The shift to the third stage is again stimulated by a change in the causal environment with resurgence of a related social problem. . . . In order to achieve the third stage, social interest, the agency must move from an internally oriented posture back to an externally oriented one . . . the thrust for delivery of service to meet the new pressing problem assumes importance (Perlmutter, 1972, pp. 109-110).

Representing the Organization and Its Interest

I have been emphasizing the social dimension of the executive's ethical responsibility as it may affect or have a bearing on the executive's administrative responsibility in and to the social organization. Assuming increasing responsiveness on the part of the social organization to its responsibility for helping to meet the needs of its community and society, and the role of the executive in relation to that responsibility, the fact remains that the executive is morally required—it is the executive's ethical responsibility—to relate to, and deal with the organization on the basis of its existing status and experience, and on the basis of the executive's assigned and ascribed responsibility in relation to both. Whatever the ultimate responsibility of the executive in and to the social organization, and in relation to the broader social responsibility of both the organization and the executive, the executive has ethical responsibility to the organization as it is and as it functions. One of the forms which executive responsibility to the organization takes is that of representing it as such, not simply its interests. As administrator, the executive is morally obligated to represent the social organization accurately as well as loyally, even as change in it may be contemplated, addressed, facilitated, and initiated. The provision in the NASW Code of Ethics that the social worker "should distinguish clearly between statements and actions made as a private individual and as a representative of . . . an organization or group" (1979) applies to executives in general.

The executive advances the interests of the organization as they are, pending changes in it should they be indicated in the context of social responsibility, and even in the context of organizational purpose and function. And the executive makes clear when actions are taken in the organization's behalf and when they are not. This is the executive's ethical responsibility even if other ethical responsibilities concurrently apply, which means that deviations from it are not supposed to occur with equanimity but require justification and accounting.

Confidentiality at the Administrative Level

An analogue to the social worker's responsibility to clients is the executive's responsibility to keep the organization's secrets. There is intelligence to which an executive becomes privy because of the very nature of the executive's position and function in the organization. The executive is bound by the principle of confidentiality in relation to the organization just as much as the social worker is in relation to a direct service client. The relevant consideration for the executive, very much like that for the social worker, is not simply that an unauthorized revelation might conceivably affect the fate and well-being of the organization adversely, but that it might offend the preferences of the organization, however mistaken they may be. Whatever social or professional motive might move the executive to reveal organizational confidences—as noble and altruistic as it might be—whatever the executive's reasons for revealing the confidences, the executive is ethically bound to avoid doing so. Those confidences are accessible to the executive only because of the executive's relationship to the organization and responsibility in it. Both the relationship and the responsibility represent a risk to the organization and an opportunity for the executive to inflict the consequences of that risk on the organization. Confidentiality becomes in effect a precondition for the executive's loyal and devoted service to the organization. The executive must be worthy of the trust this implies.

This does not mean that such loyalty and devotion are infinitely capacious. Neither does it mean that as an ethical principle the expectation is readily dispensable, even in the interest of what may be regarded as superseding values or ethical responsibilities, including even those to which the organization itself is committed. To neglect it is to deviate from ethical responsibility and at the very least the reasons for doing so must be demonstrably compelling—a matter of life and death perhaps or something quite close to that. The judgment would then be not that the deviation was ethical; only that under the pressure of extreme circumstances it was understandable.

The Interests of Social Organizations and the Interests of Others

Conscientious executives sometimes have a problem in choosing between the organization's interests and the interests of others to whom they also feel ethical responsibility. The stakes in justice and equity for others, for example, sometimes impress them as being inordinately high—high enough to betray the organization. They sometimes feel compelled to "blow the whistle;" nor do they, as a result, always enjoy a hero's welcome, our society's norms being what they are sometimes. Nevertheless, they cannot always contain themselves or their zeal for justice and equity. Occasionally, an organization's actions border on, if not cross over into, the grossly illegal (that is, criminal) and unethical, with manifestly destructive and discriminatory consequences for innocent and unsuspecting clients and others. An executive may indeed "blow the whistle." For such a choice to be made by the executive, the loyalty and devotion owed to the organization must be appreciably outdistanced by the contravening ethical considerations which prompt the executive to act. And considerable conviction and fortitude are required of the executive since, under such circumstances, the executive seat waxes hot and not infrequently it is pulled out from under the executive. (I am assuming of course that all less extreme alternatives have been duly explored and exhausted in the very interest of justice and equity.)

From a practical point of view, it sometimes makes sense for an executive to resort to this ultimate strategy in the attempt to effect salutary change rather than quietly withdrawing or resigning in muted protest. And, as a colleague once put it, an executive who quits in protest or disgust over some malefaction or other without attempting corrective action in the process, is often not certain whether the exit was made voluntarily via the front door, or involuntarily via the back window—figuratively speaking of course. If an executive has to go, the departure ought to be designed to serve some useful social purpose. But there should be no mistake about one thing: strictly speaking, whistle-blowing, however motivated, is unethical when it is done by the executive, just as it is when done by anybody else in the organization.

Symbolic and Practical Significance of Organizational Representation

An undercurrent issue in relation to the ethics of social work administration in all of these circumstances is whether and how the social organization is or should be represented by the executive. Representing the social organization is more than a matter of speaking for it, and representing and acting on its interests. The way in which the executive represents the organization carries symbolic as well as expressive and functional significance and consequences. In the eyes of others, inside and outside of the organization, the executive *is* the organization. Neither may be the elongated shadow of the other, but what the executive is and does is often viewed not only as *in behalf of* the organization, but *as* the organization.

The executive of a social organization often serves as the personification of the organization. When organization personnel refer to the "administration" they usually mean the executive or the collectivity of administrators. This is hardly inappropriate since, as I have emphasized, it is not organizations which act but the people in them. But the meaning in this usage is more extensive. In it, the executive is regarded as the embodiment of the policies, the norms, the values, the aspirations, the deficiencies, the failings, the malice, the injustices, the virtues, the ineptitudes, and so on, of the organization as a whole. And those of these characteristics which are perceived in the executive are attributed to the organization. Nor are these tendencies entirely unrealistic, although they are often charged with exaggerated affect.

The imprint of the executive is often manifest in the organization. It is also possible that some executives become socialized into the ways of the organization. When executives are "strong" leaders—decisive, efficient, systematic, etc.—the atmosphere and practices in their organizations are likely to be brisk, productive, clear. When executives are "weak" leaders—indecisive, passive, laissez-faire—the atmosphere and practices in their organizations are likely to be disquieting, egocentrically and competitively oriented. When executives are authoritarian leaders—arbitrary, secretive, inaccessible—the atmosphere and practices are likely to be tense, nervously driven, rivalrous, paternalistic.

These are not *necessary* consequences, only likely consequences, but the point to be emphasized is that in this sense of representation, ethical responsibility at the executive level is a function of the reality that executives not only represent their organizations, but are also a reflection of and on their organizations. Executives therefore carry ethical responsibility of rather gigantic proportions which extend beyond the reasonable boundaries of occupational responsibility, and tend to infringe on their very persons and privacy.

Human service practitioners sacrifice a large measure of autonomy for the privilege of professional practice—a sacrifice implicit in the very definition of profession as oriented to human service, and as premised on social values. The sacrifice is also explicit as well as implicit in the codes of ethics by which they are usually bound. Executives of social organizations lose a perhaps larger measure of autonomy when they assume the mantle of administrative office. They are certainly not free to do as they please in office, but neither are they free to do as they please out of office.

Not only is the morality of their administrative practice affected, but the morality of their personal practices as well, as unjust as this may seem on the face of it—for human beings are entitled to their share of independence and privacy even if they do happen to be executives of social organizations. Executives of social organizations are obliged, as a matter of ethical responsibility, to consider the effect on their organizations of their behavior off as well as on the job. Whether they will it or not, they do serve as symbols of their organizations and everything that those symbols represent. An additional burden on executives is their valuation of what the organizations exist to do, and for whom. On the shoulders of the executives rest what they may regard as urgent programs and services for many persons in critical need of them. Executives with half a conscience can hardly take lightly such risks to those programs and services, and to the capacity of their organizations to provide them, as their private, let alone official conduct may pose.

Executives may, of course, also be concerned about their own necks, but a response to that type of concern or any other self-interest is hardly a response to ethical responsibility. The responsibility of executives as organizational symbols stretches much farther than their necks.

It would appear to be unnecessary to emphasize the caution which executives are required to exercise when speaking and acting in and for their organizations, since their ethical responsibility in those connections flows directly from defined administrative responsibility. It is necessary, however, to emphasize the ethical responsibility of executives to employ similar caution in their activities unrelated to their organizational functions, whether as moonlighting practitioners, or as volunteers, or simply as private citizens. They must feel ethically compelled to do nothing anywhere to demean their office or embarrass their organizations.

Ethics requires of executives that they avoid any conduct, position, or association which might conceivably reflect adversely on the dignity of their administrative positions, or on their trustworthiness and reliability in those positions. This includes not only unethical, illegal, or unseemly conduct—like consorting with gangsters, or frequenting opium dens, or becoming inebriated, or gambling away huge sums of money, or chasing after women. It includes any other activity which is rated low in respectability in their communities, and especially low in relation to conduct regarded in those communities as becoming administrators of well-regarded social organizations. An executive who is a lawyer, for example, and is contractually free to practice law outside the organization, cannot feel free to undertake the defense of a shady underworld figure who earns his keep by doing precisely the kind of thing that the executive's organization has been created to prevent—like selling drugs to adolescents; this despite the ethics of legal practice which presumably assures every person the availability of competent defense. Neither can a social worker who is an executive of a social organization feel free to take part-time employment as a construction site night watchman, as financially strapped as the executive might be, and as lenient as the organization's rules might be about extra-organizational employment. This is not to discredit night watchmen but to stress the ethical responsibility of the executive to consider the effect of such employment on the organization and the executive's task in it.

A question might be raised about the very assumption of extra-organizational duties in the first place, especially remunerative ones, regardless of their social standing and their organizational impact, since it is the executive's ethical responsibility to be entirely available to the employing organization, to give it full and undivided loyalty and attention. To add an example of what may be an alarmingly growing practice, it would certainly be unethical for a social organization executive who is a social worker, for example, to engage in private professional practice on the premises of the organization, and perhaps even off those premises, although about this there is likely to be more controversy.

The issue for ethics of extra-organizational employment is both a quantitative and qualitative one. It is a scalar issue in that it affects the level of the executive's outside activity—how it ranks socially and occupationally in relation to the executive's position and authority in the organization, and in relation to the purposes and functions of the organization itself. And it is a functional issue in that it affects the nature and effect of the executive's activity in relation to the needs and expectations of the organization and the executive's job in it. Would it be an embarrassment to the organization for the executive to earn a pittance breaking batteries in a junkyard, and to do so under the supervision of an ignorant and offensive lout? And would the executive have sufficient energy and creativity left to do the administrative work required in the organization? The private life of the executive remains private unless and until it affects the executive's job and the organization demonstrably, but many things do affect both. The organization is of course not exempt from the responsibility to treat and compensate the executive adequately enough to make these detours unnecessary—but that is another story.

The Executive and Labor-Management Relations

As a final consideration, though not an exhaustive one, I should like to consider briefly the executive's role in labor-management relations in the social organization. The executive of a social organization is duty-bound—it is the executive's ethical responsibility as it can be readily inferred from the definition of administrative responsibility—to provide for the organization's material interests when participating in collective bargaining sessions and in other labor-management transactions. This includes transactions with union representatives who are identified with the same profession as the executive. Despite the executive's collegial relationship with those representatives, the executive has to be clear that, administratively, primary loyalty is owed to the organization. Nevertheless, this does not legitimate unethical conduct, or even discourteous conduct in relation to those colleagues.

For effective labor-management relations, representatives of labor are obliged to represent labor and representatives of management are obliged to represent management. There is little room for the kind of objectivity and empathy which are required for social work service. Professional discipline is inappropriate. On the other hand, some of the principles of interpersonal relations which are characteristic of social work practice and administration may help to accomplish the ends of labor-management relations without violating some of the more sacred principles of social work practice (Levy, 1964, pp. 115-116).

Some of the guides to ethical conduct appropriate for social organization executives in labor-management relations are suggested in the NASW Code of Ethics in the section on "The Social Worker's Ethical Responsibility to Colleagues," for example: "Respect, Fairness, and Courtesy—The social worker should treat colleagues with respect, courtesy, fairness and good faith" (1979). I remember a social agency executive who identified himself as a social worker and who, in the midst of a rather tension-ridden collective bargaining session with the representatives of a social workers' union, denigrated the work of the social workers on the agency staff, declaring that their professional function as such was dispensable, unproductive, and devoid of redeeming social value. The executive's purpose, consistent with his administrative ethics, was no doubt to conserve the agency's financial resources, and to limit the cost to the agency of any contract at which the parties might arrive. On the other hand, his outburst was hardly a manifestation of the respect, fairness, courtesy, and good faith ethically due his professional colleagues. Moreover, his impetuous tirade was a manifest violation of the concept, also contained in the NASW Code of Ethics, regarding what is described in it as "Maintaining the integrity of the profession," a provision included under the category, "The Social Worker's Ethical Responsibility to the Social Work Profession" (1979).

Even if such a provision for the guidance of executives in their relationships to others in any and all circumstances, labor-management relations included, were not codified, it could readily be assumed or ascribed to them as the ethical responsibility not to foul their own professional nest, as it were, or, more affirmatively, to facilitate the effective functioning of their profession in society in order to serve such useful social purposes as the profession might be able to serve.

In short and in sum, the executive of a social organization has extensive ethical responsibility to the organization, but not so much as to justify any and all offenses to others in the process, and not so much as is entirely inconsiderate of such ethical responsibility as is due to others, and to the community and society in general.

REFERENCES

Abouzeid, Kamal M., and Weaver, Charles N. "Social Responsibility in the Corporate Goal Hierarchy," in *Readings in Management 79/80: Annual Editions* (Service Dock, Guilford, Ct.: Dushkin Publishing Group) 260-265. Reprint from *Business Horizons*, June, 1978.

Blumenthal, W. Michael. "Rx for Reducing the Occasion of 'Corporate Sin,'" in *Readings in Management 79/80: Annual Editions* (Service Dock, Guilford, Ct.: Dushkin Publishing Group) 270-273. Reprint from *S.A.M. Advance Management Journal,* Winter, 1977.

Business Week. "How Companies React to Ethics Crisis," February 9, 1976.

Drucker, Peter F. *People and Performance: The Best of Peter Drucker on Management* (New York: Harper's College Press, 1977).

Gummer, Burton. "Life at the Top: Current Research on Organizational Leadership": *Notes from the Management Literature, Administration in Social Work,* 3 (1979), 359-365.

Levy, Charles S. "Labor-Management Relations in the Jewish Community Center," *Journal of Jewish Communal Service,* 41 (1964), 114-123.

Levy, Charles S. "Personal Versus Professional Values: The Practitioner's Dilemmas," *Clinical Social Work Journal,* 4 (1976), 110-120.

Lewis, Harold. "Management in the Nonprofit Social Service Organization," *Child Welfare,* 54 (1975), 615-623.

Miringoff, Marc L. *Management in Human Service Organizations* (New York: Macmillan, 1980).

National Association of Social Workers. Code of Ethics, adopted by the NASW Delegate Assembly, November 18, 1979 (see Appendix).

Nelson, Daniel and Campbell, Stuart. "Taylorism Versus Welfare Work in American Industry: H. L. Gantt and the Bancrofts," *The Business History Review,* 46 (1972), 1-16.

Perlmutter, Felice. "A Theoretical Model of Social Agency Development," *Social Casework,* 50 (1969), 467-473.

Perlmutter, Felice. "Systems Theory and Organization Change: A Case Study," *Sociological Inquiry,* 42 (1972), 109-122.

Reinharth, Leon. "The Missing Ingredient in Organization Theory, *Readings in Management 79/80: Annual Editions* (Service Dock, Guilford, Ct.: Dushkin Publishing Group), 30-34. Reprint from *SAM Advanced Management Journal,* Winter, 1978.

Rowse, A. L., Ed. *The Annotated Shakespeare: The Tragedies and Romances* (New York: Clarkson N. Potter, 1978) Vol. III.

Silk, Leonard and Vogel, David. *Ethics and Profits: The Crisis of Confidence in American Business* (New York: Simon and Schuster, 1976).

Simon, Herbert A., Smithburg, Donald W., and Thompson, Victor A. *Public Administration* (New York: Alfred A. Knopf, 1958).

Stein, Harold, Ed. *Public Administration and Policy Development: A Case Book* (New York: Harcourt, Brace, 1952).

Titmuss, Richard M. *Social Policy* (New York: Pantheon, 1974).

Warner, W. Keith and Havens, A. Eugene. "Goal Displacement and the Intangibility of Organizational Goals," *Administrative Science Quarterly,* 12 (1968), 539-555.

VII. THE EXECUTIVE
AND THE ORGANIZATION BOARD

Thus far I have discussed the nature of ethical responsibility as it applies to administrative practice in social organizations. I have considered some of the ways in which administrative ethics may be distinguished from other morally founded behavioral expectations and some of the reasons for, and consequences of that distinction. I have suggested that some of these expectations apply to non-administrative as well as administrative staff of social organizations. The expectations in each case are associated with 1) the functions which individuals perform in the organizations, 2) the relationships which those functions occasion, and 3) the risks to others and to the organizations which are generated and made possible *because* of the responsibilities which they carry, the functions they perform, and the relationships in which they engage in the performance of those functions.

Every organizational responsibility of every person in the social organization, I have emphasized, represents an opportunity, on one hand, to perform a function in and for the organization and, on the other, to neglect that function. Every exposure of every person, resource, reputation, and other material or intangible thing of value in and to the organization, and to others affected by the organization, also represents an opportunity to serve a productive social purpose, or an unproductive and even destructive end. Ethics, therefore, includes not only the prevention or avoidance of that which it is occupationally "wrong" to do in any organizational capacity, but also the obligation to do that which it is occupationally "right" to do according to the highest moral standards of organizational conduct.

I have indicated, in various ways and in various connections, that there is much that is common, by way of administrative ethics as well as administrative practice, to profit-making and social organizations alike. However, the social purposes of social organizations—whether these be to provide sensitive services affecting the health, the relationships, the emotional well-being, and so on, of persons, or to arrange and organize programs and activities for the expression of their interests, for their personal growth and development, or for other common pursuits—the purposes of social organizations, and the ultimate ends to which they address their efforts, are appreciably different in significant ways from those of business and industrial organizations. Therefore, the ethics prescribed for the personnel of social organizations differs from that of business and industrial organizations, if not so much in substance then in operation and application.[1]

This, I have insisted, does not mean that the ethics of one is superior to the other. At the same time, the constraints on the personnel of social organizations, and the expectations ascribed to them, do appear to be greater. Consumer response, competition, and profit considerations tend to be more serviceable as behavioral constraints in business and industrial organizations than they are in social organizations. To the extent, on the other hand, that ethics has been codified and enforced for those occupations which operate in social organizations, to that extent the ethics of those occupations serves as a limitation on the organizational conduct of personnel in social organizations.

I have begun, in the last two chapters, to concentrate on the ethical responsibility of executives of social organizations. Although administrative responsibility is dispersed among a number of organization personnel, either by job definition, or delegation, or even organizational circumstances—depending upon size and scope of organizational structure and activities—ultimate administrative responsibility, and hence ultimate ethical responsibility, is generally lodged in or ascribed to the executive as the chief administrator.

Volunteer leaders of a social organization—board members of voluntary social organizations, for example—are hardly exempt from ethical responsibility but, in premises and accountability as well as in operation, their ethical responsibility does differ from that of the executive. The ethical responsibility of volunteer leaders is primarily a function of the relationship of the social organization to its present and prospective clientele and its community rather than their own personal relationship to either. As Schmidt put it:

> The members of a social agency's board of directors are the elected or appointed representatives of those citizens who have associated themselves in support of the agency. They are entrusted with the power of trusteeship over the agency. They are the link between society as a whole and those people being served by the agency (1959, p. 40).

The Executive's Relationship to the Social Organization Board

We now come to one of the loci of ethical responsibility which, perhaps more closely than those already considered, approximates, at the administrative level, the professional relationships between professional practitioners and their

---

[1]Compare the following comment by Richard M. Cyert, whose essays, though emphasizing the management of universities, do contend with management issues in the broader realm of nonprofit organizations, and do consider comparisons with profit-making organizations: "I firmly believe that a single theory of management will cover all organizations. It is true that there are institutional characteristics surrounding each organization that are important for a practicing manager to know, but most should be capable of being encompassed by a good theory" (1975, pp. 174-175).

clients. The relationship of the executive to the social organization board, when there is a board or equivalent body, like that between social worker and client, for example, may be regarded as a helping relationship. However, there is a significant difference between the two relationships, despite the relevance of social work knowledge and skill to both, and despite the relevance of social work ethics to both. Whether working with clients and groups in order to provide personal services—as, for example, in a public assistance agency, or in a family service or child guidance agency—or in order to provide activity guidance—as in a social and recreational program for senior citizens, for example, or in a friendship or social group in a community center or neighborhood settlement house—the social worker's function is to help individuals and groups to attain the social ends for which they come, or for which they are referred by other institutions. The end in view may be to solve or cope with a problem in relationships among persons or between persons and their social environment; or to meet a particular need like that for funds or personal counseling. Or the reason for clients' coming or being referred to a social organization may be to enjoy interpersonal associations or cultural programs, or to develop technical, artistic, or human relations skills. Whatever they come for, and however they get there—that is, whether on their own initiative, or via institutional requirement or commitment—they come for their own sakes or in their own direct interest. They come to meet a need of their own or to meet what others perceive to be necessary, either in their own interest or in the interest of others whom they have affected or may affect, like children of abusive parents, for example, or victims of sexual violence (cf. Levy, 1967).

The "help" which social workers attempt to provide in such cases is addressed to the needs or aspirations of the individuals and groups themselves, but in each case affecting their living and social conditions, and their relationships with others. The "help" which executives attempt to provide to social organization boards and board members relates not to their needs or problems in their own right, but to their needs and problems as they may and do affect the performance of organizational functions and the fulfillment of voluntarily assumed organizational responsibilities.

Of particular significance in relation to the needs and problems of boards and board members is their ultimate bearing on clients, members, constituents, and others to whom the social organization owes institutional responsibility and whom they may affect. An executive might be concerned about the fate and well-being of individual board members, and of all of them collectively, as they plan for the social organization, make policy for it, and insure the availability of personal and material resources for the achievement of the organization's purposes, and for the implementation of the organization's functions in behalf of others. But the primary basis of the executive's concern is the occupational responsibility that the executive carries for the administration of the social organization, and the guidance and facilitation of its operation. The essential focus of the executive's helping role with board and board members is not what they may need by way of guidance and counsel for themselves, but what they may need in order to make the organization's work and operation possible and effective—including the very selection of an executive and other staff.

An obvious implication of this distinction is that the executive, whether identified as a social worker or not, applies knowledge and skill in helping others differently than does the practitioner who provides service or program guidance directly to others in their own behalf. This applies as well to principles of ethical practice. However, it is not the principles of ethical practice as such that vary but their application. The circumstances under which, the reasons for which, and the people with whom the executive performs the administrative function require the difference in application. But then every variation in circumstance, in role, in clientele, and so on, requires modulation in the approach to practice, and in the application of principles of ethical practice, both at the direct service level and at the administrative level. The purposes of the executive's interventions and practices with board and board members, as compared with those of direct service practitioners, like social workers, with their clienteles, constitute a very significant variable which calls for an appreciably different orientation to practice and ethics.

Helping a Board Member

A rather telling illustration of the way in which an executive's helping role with a board and board members may be acted out in a social organization is included in Murray Ross's book of case histories in community organization (1958). It concerns a board member of a welfare council—an organization of social organizations as it were—who assumes the chairmanship of a committee to plan an annual meeting, a task which is regarded by the council board as important to the council and to its relationship to its constituent organizations and the community as a whole. Because of personal problems, evidently, the board member does poorly enough with the task to place the annual meeting in embarrassing jeopardy (pp. 36-40).

The "case" is interesting less as an illustration of administrative practice than as an indication of the role a social organization executive may be required to play in relation to a board member in need of help. The help is not addressed to the personal problems of the board member—which seem to be real enough—but to the facilitation of his functioning in his voluntarily assumed assignment; not for his own sake but for the practical purposes of the organization. The personal effect on the board member may be quite salutary, and referral to a source of further personal assistance may even be indicated and arranged. But the focus of an executive's attention in such a case is on the specific task, on the successful performance of which the organization's reputation and effectiveness may often rest.

This case also demonstrates the need for careful discrimination on the part of the executive regarding that which it is ethically as well as administratively appropriate to do, and that which it is not appropriate to do in relation to members of an organization board. This applies whether the organization is established to perform a specific function on behalf of clients or members, or to plan, coordinate, and fund the performance of specific functions by other organizations.

Guidance for the proper choice of executive action in such a case comes as much from principles of ethical practice as from principles of administrative practice, and often more so. The issue may not be the choice of what will work best in the case—a criterion for selection which is more apt to guide executive action in profit-making organizations—but what will be valued even if it does not work. In Ross's case, for example, the most proficient and rapid course of action—time apparently having been of the essence—might very well have been to remove the board member from the chairmanship of the annual meeting committee, and to appoint someone else who was more competent and reliable. Humane and other considerations dictated otherwise, however.

It takes knowledge about human behavior to recognize the symptoms of human limitation and human need; and to appreciate the disparity between aspiration and capacity for achievement which sometimes characterizes persons even in lofty social positions. It takes administrative skill and responsibility in relation to boards and board members to be moved to do something with and about that knowledge. And it takes values and ethics to do what needs to be done with sensitivity and compassion, and to do it constructively and productively, not only in relation to the organizational mission affected, but in relation to the persons affected. The ethics of social work administration sometimes demands proportionately less emphasis on the former than the latter.

Something else is underscored in this case which has particular relevance for the ethics of social work administration. That is that the relationship between the social organization executive and the board and board members requires considerable clarity of role, and considerable sensitivity to the risks incurred as a result of that relationship. Both imply the need for ethics. And the major responsibility for meeting that need is the executive's. It is, at any rate, an occupationally-based responsibility for the executive, which it is not for the board and its members. For the board—certainly as far as its relationship to the executive is concerned—the expectation of justice, fairness, decency, and all of the other appurtenances and premises of ethics, is a function of societal and organizational norms. For the executive, this expectation is a function of occupational responsibility. For the social worker-executive it is a critical dimension of professional ethics.

The Personal Impact on Executives of the Helping Process

Ross's case is indicative of an entire array of issues in administrative ethics to which the social organization executive is subject in the fulfillment of administrative responsibility, issues which are likely to be most personal in their impact on the executive's administrative experience. Such issues, moreover, require of the executive the kind of consciousness of occupational purpose and use of self in relation to others which represents the virtual nub of practice in the human service professions.

The personal impact of which I speak refers both to the way in which social organization executives experience their relationships with boards and board members, and the way in which boards and board members experience their relationship to executives. What is for executives occupational responsibility, however, is for board and board members ingratiating beneficence. Boards and board members are not free to be unethical with impunity, but the consequence, if there is any, is avocational. For executives, on the other hand, the consequence is vocational. More awareness and conscientiousness about ethics is occupationally normative for executives, with responsibility attributable to them for the impact not only on themselves and on boards and board members, but on others as well.

> In the process of setting objectives for successful operations, ethical and moral considerations also must be taken into account, particularly the impact of management decisions on employees, the ultimate consumers of the good or service, the community, and sometimes even the nation (Benton, 1975, p. 59).

This responsibility is not the executive's alone, but the relative expectation for executives, as compared with social organization boards and board members, is frankly discriminatory. Even the unethical acts of boards and board members devolve upon executives—not in the sense that executives are responsible for those acts, but in the sense that executives are occupationally responsible for doing something about them, or preventing them in the first place if at all possible. Ralph Kramer puts into plausible perspective some of the reasons for the difference in expectation as between executives and boards and board members:

> The executive's relationship to the agency is a full-time commitment. For most of the board members,[2] it is a part-time, avocational, and segmental

---

[2]Since Kramer is discussing voluntary agencies I am not sure why he does not include *all* board members. His description would not apply to boards of many profit-making organizations, and a few non-profit organizations in which boards play a more inclusive and authoritative role.

interest. The most clear-cut difference is, of course, their relationship as employer and employee. . . . The executive has functional authority as a result of his expertise and the board members have hierarchical authority because of their formal position in the agency (1965, pp. 110, 113).

It may seem strange to attribute to the social organization executive a helping role with the board and board members when, as Kramer says, the executive is an employee of the board, and the board has hierarchical authority. William Schmidt reinforces the point when he says:

An executive who holds his appointment from a board of directors is an employee of that board. When he receives his authority and direction from the board he is accountable to it for his performance. . . . [The executive's] legal rights are superseded by what is in the best interest of his employer and of his agency (1959, pp. 57-58, 60-61).

The Executive's Power in Relation to Organization Board

In view of the premise that I myself have enunciated, namely, that power lies at the foundation of the need for ethics in social organizations (Levy, 1976, Chapter 6), the emphasis on the executive's ethical responsibility in relation to board and board members, and particularly on the implications for the executive's ethics in the helping role in relation to them, seems contradictory. It is not as contradictory as it seems, first, because the power of the board is not always what it seems to be; and, secondly, because even if it is all that it appears to be, the executive's ethical responsibility to it remains.

As for the first argument, as Kramer reminds us, using Mary Parker Follett's phrase, the board's policy adoption powers may be more an "illusion of final authority" than real

since in administering and implementing policy decisions the executive can affect their outcome and may therefore have the last word. Furthermore, it may be said that the executive, because of his skill and closer identification with the agency, tends more often to be the initiator and actually controls the process of policy formulation. His influence is manifested not only in the selection of particular issues but also in the presentation of information regarding the likely outcomes of alternative proposals presented to the board (1965, p. 113).

The truth, on the other hand, often is that executives do less initiating than anticipating—that is, executives often determine in advance what board and board members are likely to find acceptable and propose it, rather than determining what is necessary for the improvement of services and programs, for example, and then urging the board to approve it. To be fair about this, however, I should add that executives do play a number of roles which are designed to assist boards not only in doing justice to issues, but also in considering issues in the interest of doing justice (cf. Levy, 1962).

It is also true that boards often leave a great deal to executives who are then more free to do more initiating. As an executive revealed in an interview conducted for a study of the relationship between executives and social agency boards, some boards permit executives more power in this respect than others. Where board members and their families are served by an agency, for example, and are therefore more directly concerned about, and involved in, the operation and the outcomes of the agency's services, they leave less to the executive. Where, on the other hand, boards are removed from the actual services and programs of agencies, and are therefore less directly affected by agency decisions—the so-called outside or absentee boards, for example—they are less inclined to wield their assigned power, except when it comes to budgeting, raising and allocating funds (see, for example, Levy, 1973, pp. 81-84). And some boards simply defer to the executive: "We hired a professional man because we thought he could do the job, so let's let him do the job" (Levy, 1964, p. 41). So the executive may or may not have power; or may or may not resort to such power as may be delegated or be implicit in the organization's administrative function, and upon which ethical responsibility is based.

The executive may also lack the skill or the will to use that power. Ethical responsibility nevertheless applies *because* of the executive's relationship to the board; *because* of the executive's functional responsibility to the board and board's members, and responsibility in relation to the roles that board and board members play in the organization; and *because* of the risks to board, board members, organization, and others as a consequence of both the executive's relationship and responsibility to the board and board members.

As for the board's power to fire the executive which, if not made explicit, is certainly implicit in the board's power to hire the executive, again, it makes no difference as far as principles of administrative ethics are concerned, although it is sure to make a difference as far as the executive's behavior and responses to the board and board members are concerned—undoubtedly one of the more compelling reasons for the need for administrative ethics.

But even that power has been questioned. Richard Cyert acknowledges the possibility of a board's firing an organization's chief executive, but considers it quite rare, largely because members of the board may not feel competent enough to do it, or even to judge its validity. Cyert is inclined to think that the firing of an executive is more likely to be a result of pressure from organization participants than from an analysis of the organization's management (1975, p. 184). This may be one of the "technical questions" about which Clarence King said that board members may be empowered to decide, but lack the wherewithal to resolve. "They must therefore depend upon the advice of their executive or other experts" (1938, p. 20). King added, "There are administrative boards, legally possessed of great power but so weak in the quality of their membership that they are only rubber stamps for the executive" (p. 32), a possibility which itself dictates the necessity of administrative ethics in view of the valuation of self-determination in human service circles and particularly in social organizations (cf. Levy, 1982). The kind of board King describes is not likely to fire an executive under ordinary circumstances, although, as I have suggested, less ordinary circumstances do occur in which boards do use their firing power, and not always justly.

It does not matter, really, from the point of view of ascribing ethical responsibility to social organization executives, except for the implication that, if the board does have and use its power, or can if it should so choose, the executive must be aware of, and resist the influence of that power, especially if it induces what may be regarded as unethical conduct. And if the executive actually holds the balance of power over the board, whether by board default or circumstantial operation, and whatever the organizational definitions of the roles of both, the executive must be aware of, and resist the inclination to abuse that power, or to use it in an undisciplined or destructive fashion.

Independent Judgment Versus Self-Interest

The hazards for administrative ethics should be quite evident. Blau and Scott's characterization of the normative choices of action by human service practitioners in relation to their clients, with but slight modification, fits the relationship of the social organization executive and the board and board members:

> The professional's decisions are expected to be governed not by his own self-interest but by his judgment of what will serve the client's interest best. The professions are institutionalized to assure, in the ideal case, that the practitioner's self-interest suffers if he seeks to promote it at the expense of optimum service to clients.
>
> Professional service also requires, however, that the practitioner maintain independence of judgment and not permit the clients' *wishes,* as distinguished from their *interests,* to influence his decisions (1962, pp. 51-52; cf. Levy, 1976, pp. 124-126).

These amount to first principles of ethics in social work administration since they represent generalized perspectives of the executive's role in relation to the social organization board and its members. It is the executive's ethical responsibility to concentrate on the board's purposes in dealing with the board and its members; to help the board and its members implement their charge as trustees of the community and the organization's present and prospective membership and clientele; and to block the intrusion of extraneous needs and vested interests, whether of board members or the executive, on the performance of their functions and the fulfillment of their assigned responsibilities. This says nothing about the skill and competence which are required in order to attain these ends; only about the executive's moral obligation to address them and to do so ethically. Implied as well are the values by which the executive is guided in addressing them.

The Non-Judgmental Attitude

One of these values is that of acceptance or the "non-judgmental attitude" (Biestek, 1953). This value, and the principle of ethical practice which is founded upon it, deprive the social organization executive of the human right of ordinary mortals to pass judgment on others, and to permit that judgment to influence their actions in relation to those upon whom they pass judgment. Not that these are such desirable inclinations. But persons who are not executives, or who otherwise do not suffer the affliction of a helping relationship in behalf of others, are free to have and to coddle those inclinations—as long as they break no laws, or offend no enforceable moral strictures in the process. They might be subject to group censure as being unfair, but they are not bound by the kind of occupational commitment to cease and desist that executives are in their relationship to their boards and board members.

Executives are not obliged to like such a commitment, which they are not likely to do when they find boards and board members mean-spirited and malicious, but they are obliged to resist any tendency to evade that commitment. The non-judgmental attitude in dealing with boards and board members, at least, is reasonably prescribed as a component of the ethics of social work administration.

The Limitations of Boards and Board Members

Clarence King realistically acknowledges the fact that boards are frequently an impediment to task achievement, and are often self-perpetuating and controlled by disproportionate concentrations of power; hardly less a fact than what he regards as the perverse motivations of some board members in accepting their positions on boards. But, perhaps surprisingly, King is not pessimistic about these things, for he goes on to say that "mixed motives do not necessarily hamper the work" (1938, p. 17). And Arnold Auerbach offers the "thesis" that *"there is no basic contradiction between the aspirations for power, prestige, and recognition and dedicated devotion to agency goals"* (1961, p. 71). Auerbach does suggest that "the difficulty comes only in the way these motivations are sometimes expressed and in the manner in which we as professionals [i.e., executives] have handled them" (p. 17). These reassurances only signify that nothing much need be lost organizationally when the interests and inclinations of board members are not entirely in harmony with the purposes, functions, and effective operation of the organization.

The point at issue as far as administrative ethics is concerned is that the executive takes board members as they are. It is the privilege of board members to be as they are. The executive does not enjoy the same privilege, not ethically at any rate. The executive deals with them—as the NASW Code of Ethics puts it—"in accordance with the highest standards of professional integrity and impartiality" (1979). If practitioners are to be judged on the basis of their occupational acts and not on the basis of their motives, as I have suggested (Levy, 1980), then certainly board members who are not vocationally bound by codified occupational ethics—not in their board capacities, at least—should not be judged by executives on that basis. To bridge two ideological concepts, the executive *values* board members in their own right, and *helps* them to fulfill their organizational responsibility.

Helping board members includes calling attention to values and responsibilities related to, or affecting the work and goals of the social organization, as unpleasant as the consequences in board disapproval or personal responses might prove to be. It takes the pressure of ethical responsibility for executives to overcome their fears and doubts in relation to their comfort and self-interest, both of which might be jeopardized by their incurring the displeasure of boards or board members. And there is also the risk that an executive's attempt to counteract organizationally subversive board preferences might not even work. But the attempt must be made if the executive is to be ethical. Joseph Steiner also seems to be concerned about the negative consequences, for organizational progress, of board deficiences along these lines, but nevertheless implies executive responsibility when he says:

> A common shortcoming of policy-making groups is their failure to acknowledge the importance of value premises. When these premises are avoided in policy-making discourse, they frequently become conflicting underlying agendas that effectively block progress (1976, p. 80).

Helping the Board to Fulfill Organization Objectives

Whether the result is blocked progress or not, it is incumbent upon the executive to remind the board of neglected values and anything else that merits consideration in the ethical as well as effective performance of the board's and the organization's functions, policy-making and policy-implementing functions included.

The executive's interventions in the fulfillment of ethical responsibility may be addressed simply to the adherence to avowed organizational intentions; or to adherence in a nondiscriminatory manner should a plan for implementing those intentions result in an intended or circumstantial deprivation of client or staff opportunities. A social agency camp, for example, was established to serve elderly persons whose income was pitifully limited. Partly because of financial pressures, but primarily because camp policy inevitably led to applications from a large proportion of non-white persons, the board met one day to revise the application procedures and fees, and to redefine eligibility criteria so that what board members regarded as a preferable ethnic distribution of the camp's clientele would result.

The members of the board seemed to be of one mind about these modifications in policy and procedures, so much so that the executive could not persuade them, with data and reminders of the camp's original purpose, that their actions were misguided. The board stuck to its resolve with virtual unanimity. The executive mulled the matter over quickly, very mindful of the risk he might have to take, and finally declared himself: the modifications which the board had just approved, he said, were inconsistent with the board's own commitments regarding the camp's purpose and clientele. It was those commitments which had influenced his acceptance of the appointment as executive. Now that they had evidently been cast aside, he could not in good conscience continue in the position.

The board did reverse itself—which was hardly the unhappy ending that the executive might have expected. However, his action was inspired by the ethical responsibility he felt obliged to fulfill—to both the organization and its intended clientele, for whom the proposed changes were, in the executive's eyes, discriminatory. Fortunately for him, the action worked, but as ethical responsibility it had to be taken whether it worked or not.

Representativeness of Board

The interventions of a social organization executive, in the fulfillment of ethical responsibility, might also be addressed to the very composition of a board, and to its representativeness in relation to the organization's purposes and clientele. If what a recent study of boards of directors in social organizations says about boards is generally true, then administrative ethics would dictate executive initiative in doing something about it, for the study reports that:

> Boards are charged with not being broadly representative of the public, with being out of touch with the people they propose to serve, and unresponsive to the problems of the day. Their membership, it is charged, tends to be limited to older, upper-income, professional employer and managerial persons, while the clientele (or community) has little or no representation . . . much of the current self-examination by Boards of voluntary agencies has been prompted by frankly financial considerations (The Greater New York Fund, 1974, p. xvi).

This need not be entirely or exclusively true to warrant an executive's concern and intervention. To the extent that it is true of a social organization board, it does suggest the values by which the executive must feel guided. What an executive is occupationally moved to value in relation to a social organization board's decisions and actions, the executive is morally obliged to express in specific actions (cf. Levy, 1979, p. 2).

The social organization executive "keeps the board honest" by checking board actions which purport to be responsive to the right of clients and consumers to be represented in board deliberations, or at least to have their needs and interests affirmatively and accurately represented. The executive intervenes to help board members determine whether their actions are truly so responsive, and introduces questions and considerations designed to make them more so when they are not. If advisory groups, for example, are not truly advisory in this respect, and serve only as a way of defusing restless clienteles, it is up to the executive, as a matter of administrative ethics, to tell the board so, and to influence the board as much as possible to make such groups as advisory as they are supposed to be, if not even more influential than that.

Honesty with clientele is not only the executive's direct responsibility, but also an indirect responsibility in relation to the social organization board. When the board is not entirely honest with organization clients, the executive does something about it (cf. Levy, 1970).

King poses a rather subtle issue in ethics when he asks whether the executive should "shrewdly manipulate" the organization board into "making the 'right' decisions" (1938, p. 53). On one hand, the executive is obliged to contemplate the ethics of a decision itself. On the other hand, the executive is obliged to contemplate the ethics of the instrumentality employed to get the decision considered and to implement it once taken. Not all means are ethically acceptable in relation to even socially desirable ends. These are the proverbial "wheels within wheels" which complicate the ethics of social work administration but which are essential for the executive to conjure with.

Process and Substance in Board Operation

Ethics requires of social organization executives as much substance as form of approach to work with boards and board members. Social workers who are executives tend to be infatuated with process, which is of course important in administrative practice, and often the major locus of administrative ethics. That is, it is often in process—what goes on among people, their impact and effect on one another in relation to what they come together to accomplish and to do, and how they go about doing it—it is often in process that ethics, and issues in ethics, are most manifest. However, process is insufficient, as is an executive's preoccupation with process, if it does not serve the purposes that a board is charged to serve in behalf of the social organization. John Wax puts this very well, I think:

> Decision-making is more than process; there is important content also. The overt, conscious, or explicit material consists primarily of information. . . . [These are] the factual premises in decision-making. The second type of content . . . may be covert, unconscious, less visible, and less discussable, or it may be explicit, philosophical, and ideological (1971, pp. 285-286).

Facilitating the Board's Work

The executive needs more than style and finesse in working with the organization board, as useful as these may be. The executive also needs homework—preparation, facts, principles, etc.—in order to provide more than tears and exhortations, and sounds and alarums. These may also be regarded as administrative responsibility, and the prerequisites of sound and effective administrative practice. But it is ethical responsibility as well.[3] The board relies on the executive to provide, or provide for, what it may need to do its work thoroughly and well, and to make well-founded decisions. These are ultimately the board's responsibilities, but their facilitation is part of the executive's work. To be ill-equipped for it is analogous to the failure to have or to acquire the competence to perform the professional functions for which a professional practitioner assumes responsibility, an expectation for which the NASW Code of Ethics makes explicit provision (1979).

King talks about the kind of zeal of social organization boards for perfectly valid and noble causes, which may become excessive and have to be curbed (1938, p. 18). Executives may also be afflicted by such zeal, especially when they happen to be socially committed human service practitioners who espouse important social causes which they perceive to affect disproportionately the health and well-being of already deprived and disadvantaged persons. They may resort to questionable strategies in serving those causes.

---

[3]"Executives who are occupying key administrative posts have a trust to increase their knowledge and sharpen their skills by every means possible. Herein lies the key to the improvement of social services" (Schmidt, 1959, p. 9). The idea of trust itself has ethical connotations, but when Schmidt adds the reference to the improvement of social services, he seems to be stressing its pragmatic connotations. At the same time, there is implicit in this reference the duty owed by executives to those who are affected, or who may be affected by social services. The executive looks beyond the board, and the relationship between them, to others to whom ethical responsibility is also owed. Again, the concern is not merely what will work better administratively, but what it is the moral obligation of the executive to do, although in this case as in many others the two do happen to coincide. Not infrequently, however, they do not.

Interpersonal Relationships in Boards

There are ethical limits to be considered in resorting to such strategies. Secret alignments with sympathetic board members, for example, are questionable. If that is the case with legitimate causes which are compatible with the functions and purposes of the social organization for which the board acts, it is certainly the case with aspirations extraneous to the organization's purposes and functions, or in conflict with them.

Personal alignments of executives with board members who are already pitched in conflict with other board members, for the sole or primary purpose of rallying support for themselves or their preferences, are clearly unethical. And yet they are sometimes resorted to by social organization executives intent on attaining their ends, their personal comfort, or security in their jobs.

Subjective Bases of Executive Actions

A similar effect is possible when executives have strong preferences regarding persons who are candidates for offices on the board, or, more's the pity, persons who are not candidates but whom executives would like to see in office for the simple reason that they might be easier to work with, or perhaps safer. This, too, is hardly ethical, not for some obscure moral reason, but because executives have both opportunity and responsibility to expedite and even influence sound and proficient selections of officers and board members, on the basis of objective and factually relevant criteria.

Executives may have social aspirations or even material ones—personal wealth, for example—which may move them to seek and exploit personal relationships with board members for personal gain (board members sometimes know a lot about investments) or in order to curry favor with them. (The manipulative character of such efforts may be suggested by the expressions sometimes used to describe them: *cultivating* or *courting* board members.) If it is not too indiscreet to mention it, I have known of an executive or two whose jobs seemed to hang on the rather thin thread of an illicit affair with a board president. Whatever the motivation, social organization executives are ethically bound to maintain strictly professional relationships with board members, as convenient and cozy as their lives may be made by more personal relationships. Affective or emotional neutrality (that is, objectivity and not hard-nosed detachment) is more than a sociological phenomenon. It is an ethical necessity which applies to the relationship between executive and board members as it does to the relationship between human service practitioners and their clients or patients, although the functional nature of each of these relationships does affect the nature of its operation. In a way—under ordinary circumstances at any rate—the relationship between executives and board members of social organizations tends to be a bit more relaxed and easy-going, give or take the impact of the differences in social position between them, since board members are not coming to the executives for help with sensitive personal or social problems. There is more the spirit of working together on common concerns in relation to, and on behalf of others. But, perhaps, that is a good reason for underscoring the need for caution on the part of social organization executives. It is easier to forget oneself under such circumstances (cf. Wilensky and Lebeaux, 1958, pp. 300-301).[4]

I have been placing the primary burden of ethical responsibility on the social organization executive, largely because of the executive's occupational status from which derives an entire set of occupational responsibilities, and premises for them, both of which are distinguishable from those which affect boards and board members. Still, executives of social organizations are not always in full control of their relationship to board and board members; nor are boards and board members always passive enough participants to permit executives much initiative in relating to them.

Limiting Board Autonomy

As privileged as boards and board members are in their relationship to executives, as compared with the executives, it is nevertheless incumbent on executives to attempt to draw boundaries, or at least to suggest them, around the autonomy of boards and board members. Boards and board members are entitled to the pleasure of their associations, and even to their personal animosities. They are entitled to their satisfactions, and even to their perverse motivations and aspirations but, as Auerbach put it, "no matter how strong the need for power and prestige, no group or individual can justify an agency policy on that basis alone" (1961, p. 72).

Perhaps optimistically, Auerbach goes on to say, "the stated social and ethical objectives of our agencies themselves are powerful guiding and controlling factors" (p. 72). These objectives may or may not be as guiding and controlling as he seems to hope, but they are certainly factors that executives are

---

[4]Sometimes the circumstances are not so "ordinary." There is occasionally so much tension between board and executive that they act more like adversaries than the partners they are often presumed to be (e.g., Brodsky, 1957). This is usually symptomatic of more serious problems between the two which do not bode well for either the relationship or the organization. Most often it does not bode very well for the executive either. It should be obvious, by the way, that I am not presuming to apply these observations to corporate industrial boards and executives, despite an occasional similarity. That, again, is quite another story, as any account, fictitious or otherwise, of the machinations of the executive suite will attest. The relationships are different, and the functions are different. And the rules are also different.

morally obligated to represent in working with boards and board members, and to do so without fear or favor. On the other hand, boards and board members—especially prestigious, powerful, affluent, and influential ones—can be intimidating, especially for executives who originate in lower socio-economic circles, and for executives who do not feel secure in their jobs. Ethics nevertheless requires executives to be on guard against the operation of their personal biases and defensiveness.

Although the ethics of boards and board members—as limited as it is in comparison with that of executives—is not the subject of this discussion, I must add that, as between board and executive, it takes two to tango ethically. This hardly legitimates unethical conduct on the part of an executive. On the other hand, a board should not be surprised by the emergence of the "evil inclination" of an executive subjected to unethical conduct. As in any relationship, when one of the parties to it is ethical to a fault and the other is not ethical at all, the former is seriously disadvantaged. This danger affects especially those social organizations in which boards carry, and are inclined to exploit, considerable authority and power over the executive (e.g., Smith, 1955).

Administrative Ethics as Opportunity

This is unfortunately a rather negative slant on the ethics of social work administration. Ethics need hardly be a militaristic type of offensive maneuver. It is really an opportunity which is best guided by the principles of ethical practice commonly associated with relationships and idealized practice in human service professions. The ethical executive respects the dignity of board members, and strives to preserve it. The ethical executive respects the privacy of board members, and is disciplined enough to avoid infringements upon it. The ethical executive safeguards the confidences shared by board members in the course of their work together. The ethical executive does not "treat" (as social worker, for example) board members since such a treatment relationship is not compatible with the kind of working relationship required for board members and executives, and is likely to conflict with it since the two relationships are guided and affected by disparate goals.

Even more positively, the ethics of social work administration represents an opportunity both to influence the ethics of board operation and to make possible the maximum development of board members, *as* board members—which is to say, never at the expense of the organizational tasks to be accomplished, or functions to be performed, but as a possible consequence of both. This may be the highest form of occupational and administrative respect, for it reflects a valuation of board members as ends in themselves and not merely as instruments of organizational achievement.

REFERENCES

Auerbach, Arnold J. "Aspirations of Power People and Agency Goals," *Social Work*, 6 (1961), 66-73.

Benton, Lewis. Introduction to Part II, "The Discussion," in Richard M. Cyert, *The Management of Non Profit Organizations (With Emphasis on Universities)* (Lexington, Mass.: D. C. Heath, 1975).

Biestek, Felix P. "The Non-judgmental Attitude," *Social Casework*, 34 (1953), 235-239.

Blau, Peter M. and Scott, W. Richard. *Formal Organizations: A Comparative Approach* (San Francisco: Chandler Publishing, 1962).

Brodsky, Irving. *Manual for Board Members: A Guide for Service* (New York: National Jewish Welfare Board, 1957).

Cyert, Richard M. *The Management of Non profit Organizations (With Emphasis on Universities)* (Lexington, Mass.: D. C. Heath, 1975).

The Greater New York Fund. *Boards of Directors: A Study of Current Practices in Board Management and Board Operations in Voluntary Hospital, Health and Welfare Organizations* (New York: Oceana Publications, 1974.)

Kramer, Ralph M. "Ideology, Status, and Power in Board-Executive Relationships," *Social Work*, 10 (1965), 107-114.

Levy, Charles S. "Client Self-Determination: Keystone or Millstone of Social Work Ethics," Aaron Rosenblatt and Diana Waldfogel, Eds. *Handbook of Clinical Social Work* (San Francisco: Jossey-Bass, Publishers, 1982).

Levy, Charles S. *Education and Training for the Fundraising Function* (New York: The Lois and Samuel Silberman Fund for the Bureau for Careers in Jewish Service, 1973).

Levy, Charles S. "The Executive and the Agency Board," *Journal of Jewish Communal Service*, 38 (1962), 234-248.

Levy, Charles S. *The Executive and the Jewish Community Center Board* (New York: National Jewish Welfare Board, 1964).

Levy, Charles S. "Personal Motivation as a Criterion in Evaluating Social Work Practice," *Social Casework*, 61 (1980), 541-547.

Levy, Charles S. "Power through Participation: The Royal Road to Social Change," Points and Viewpoints, *Social Work*, 15 (1970), 105-108.

Levy, Charles S. "The 'Problem' in the Social Work 'Problem-Solving' Process," *Journal of Jewish Communal Service*, 43 (1967), 304-311.

Levy, Charles S. *Social Work Ethics* (New York: Human Sciences Press, 1976).

Levy, Charles S. *Values and Ethics for Social Work Practice*, Continuing Education Series, No. 11 (Washington, D. C.: National Association of Social Workers, 1979).

National Association of Social Workers. Code of Ethics, Adopted by the NASW Delegate Assembly, November 18, 1979 (see Appendix).

Ross, Murray G. *Case Histories in Community Organization* (New York: Harper and Brothers, 1958).

Schmidt, William D. *The Executive and the Board in Social Welfare* (Cleveland, Ohio: Howard Allen, 1959).

Smith, Harvey L. "Two Lines of Authority: The Hospital's Dilemma," in Gerald D. Bell, ed., *Organizations and Human Behavior* (Englewood Cliffs, N. J.: Prentice-Hall, 1967), 109-117.

Steiner, Joseph R. "Discourse Management: Key to Policy Development," *Journal of Sociology and Social Welfare*, 4 (1976), 73-80.

Wax, John, "Power Theory and Institutional Change," *The Social Service Review*, 45 (1971), 274-288.

Wilensky, Harold L. and Lebeaux, Charles N. *Industrial Society and Social Welfare* (New York: Russell Sage Foundation, 1958).

VIII. THE EXECUTIVE
AND THE ORGANIZATION STAFF

Cusson and Laberge-Altmejd (1977) have stated that one need only have experienced the power of another to appreciate its potential for destructiveness. And it is quite possible to underestimate the satisfaction that may be derived from wielding power over another or others, with consequences extending out to a community and even to a nation, at times by the simple use of speech or gesture.[1]

Using and Abusing Administrative Power

One's subjugation to the power of another does not always constrain one's own use and abuse of power over others in turn. There are times when, instead of identifying with the victims of abused power as a consequence *of one's own* victimization by the power of others, one commits with others the same or similar offenses.

Executives of social organizations are subject to such power as organization boards or other officials are authorized, competent, equipped, and inclined to wield, but they, in turn, have power to wield over subordinates, depending upon their own equipment and inclination and, of course, depending upon their own ethics. If boards or other officials, by virtue of their authority to hire and fire executives, can choose to keep executives unsettled and on the *qui vive,* executives, by virtue of their authority to hire and fire members of the organization staff—although sometimes, but not always, with the required approval of others—can do the same with them.

What executives do with the power at their disposal, beyond its use to expedite the functioning of the organization, is primarily a function of their ethics. The failure to use that power may be just as unethical as using it unjustly or excessively. But they do have the power, and there is no telling how that power may be used:

---

[1]"Il suffit d'avoir été à la merci d'hommes puissants pour savoir que l'exercice du pouvoir risque de se transformer en passion destructice. Aussi, le premier pas à faire dans une réflexion sur un tel sujet est d'éviter une erreur; celle de sous-estimer les satisfactions qu'apporte le pouvoir. 'Il ne faut pas une longue expérience,' écrivait Jean-Jacques Rousseau, 'pour sentir combien il est agréable d'agir par les mains d'autrui et de n'avoir besoin que de remuer la langue pour faire mouvoir l'univers.' Le simple fait de voir d'autres hommes agir selon notre volonté est gratifiant. Et si, par surcroît, l'obéissance nous permet de réaliser nos projects, ce pouvoir nous apporte une double satisfaction" (Cusson and Laberge-Altmejd, 1977, p. 238).

> The administrator wields power; he has the capability of influencing the behavior of others. This power is vested in the administrator because he occupies a particular position, the nature of which requires the exercise of authority to direct the work of others. The sources of administrative power . . . are impersonal and objective. . . . A generous admixture of subjective elements, however, frequently contaminates administrative behavior (Berliner, 1971, p. 562).

Executives could hardly do their jobs without "the power and right to act in behalf of the whole agency" but that power "is not arbitrary personal power but functional authorization which comes with the job. It is authority with others rather than over them (Trecker, 1950, p. 98)." Although the functional authorization accorded to the executive's administrative actions differs from that accorded the actions of a social organization board, for example, and in some respects is conditioned by and dependent upon the board's authority, both the executive and the board constitute the organization's elite in relation to other organization staff members.

> Those with power impress their will on others. They have a disproportionate voice in the legislation of policy and the distribution of resources. Since an elite controls the system of sanctions they can limit choice and thereby regulate the behavior of others in the organization. Those who are not in the elite are vulnerable to tyranny because they are without "equal protection" and access to an "impartial judicial system" (Scott, 1969, p. 49).

Whether or not the non-elite person enjoys the equal protection to which Scott refers in this statement, or has access to an impartial judicial system, are variables, subject to executive manipulation. "Though executive authority is inherent in the [administrative] situation," as Trecker indicates (1950, p. 98), such deprivations for staff are not inherent in but rather are functions of how executives use that authority. Robert Presthus may be quite right about the tendencies of some executives, but need hardly be describing all or even most social organization executives when, in acknowledging the executive's control of an organization's resources, he goes on to say:

> Since his role involves coordinating and arbitrating the conflicting demands of specialists [i.e., those of the organization staff], he tends to regard them in terms of power and strategy. . . . Administrators . . . tend . . . to view human beings as instruments designed to achieve ends considered by the organization to be more important than those of any individual person. As a result, organizational values become the benchmarks for evaluating and rewarding the individual (1962, pp. 21, 25).

This is not necessarily true even of all large business and industrial organizations, in which Presthus is particularly interested, let alone of all social organizations, but it is not infrequently true, executives being the variable human beings that they are. Social organization executives are no less variable and no less human than others. Perhaps that is why some system of prescriptive ethics becomes necessary when available regulatory mechanisms are not sufficiently serviceable as social controls. And one or the other is certainly as desirable for business and industrial organizations as it is for social organizations, if not more so. The idealized culture of social organizations does make it more normative and more consistent with the values associated with the purposes and functions of social organizations.

Administrative Ethics as Practical as Well as Ideological

To emphasize the ethical dimension of administrative practice in any organization is not to imply that it is invariably impractical. On the contrary, ethics is often practical, and much of organization theory which stresses the human relations component of administrative practice is quite ethical in its connotations, though primarily considerate of its practical effects for organizational purposes (cf., for example, Argyris, 1973a).[2]

Participation by organization staff in organization decision-making may be considered both an ethical and a practical desideratum. For one thing, it seems only fair to permit and even encourage staff to share in decisions which are likely to affect them (cf. Carlton, 1976), and perhaps in other decisions as well. This may be done simply as a reflection of the human decency implicit in respecting staff's judgment, and in providing means for the expression and development of their capacities. Practically speaking, participation by organization staff in organization decision-making can be a means for reaching more enlightened decisions, and a way of increasing staff acceptance of, and cooperation in the carrying out of decisions once made. Very often, participation in decision-making is permitted and encouraged with the intent of honoring one of these motives in order to realize the other, but this can operate in either direction:

> Participative decision-making as a managerial strategy has been advocated as a means of improving both the performance and satisfaction of individuals and organizations. . . . Similar to some early job satisfaction research [which is not necessarily conclusive], participation in decision-making is viewed as an ideological imperative (i.e., in a normative sense, there are those [like Argyris] who believe that participation in decision-

---

[2]Argyris refers to his strong criticism of many human relations practices as "manipulation and control of people" (1973b, p. 253).

making should be encouraged because it is beneficial for individuals in terms of personality development) (Alutto and Acito, c. 1970, pp. 1-2).[3]

On the basis of their research, Alutto and Acito express doubts about the causal relationship between employees' opportunities for participation in organization decision-making and their attitude toward their work and their employers (cf. Alutto and Belasco, 1972). Whether or not such opportunities have practical value for organizations, they often represent conduct toward staff based on values in relation to them in their own right rather than as instruments of organizational ends, and to that extent responses to ethical responsibility. Executives can make a difference.

What are pragmatic considerations for most business and industrial organizations are or should be primarily normative and ideological ones for social organizations. They are in fact imperative ones for the ethics of social work administration, whether or not they are functional for social organizations as well.[4] The social organization executive's relationship to the organization staff becomes an obvious focal point in this connection.

The Strategic Position of Executive in Relation to Staff

The social organization executive occupies a strategically advantageous position in relation to organization staff members. Available to the executive are "power-means" with which to manipulate staff members, including physical, material, and symbolic rewards (Etzioni, 1975, p. 4). Particularly potent is what has been described as the executive's remunerative power which "is based on control over material resources and rewards through allocation of salaries and wages" (p. 5), and such additional benefits as the organization has to offer and the executive has the authority to distribute.

In summarizing conceptualizations of power as an operative factor in the

---

[3]"The Maslowian basic human needs perspective . . . suggests that . . . we [human beings] have . . . important needs which are distinctively human. . . . In effect, our needs to love and be loved, for dignity, and for self-actualization may well be used to characterize, indeed define a human being. . . . *Ethically, it is in these . . . needs that our claim to be treated—and our imperative to treat others—as persons is rooted*" (Etzioni, 1975, p. 102; emphasis supplied). "A recognition of individual human dignity . . . is now implicit to a large degree in organizations of all kinds. . . . Employee satisfaction and welfare have become important values" (Pfiffner and Sherwood, 1960, pp. 9, 11).

[4]"Much of the research and speculation on behavior in organizations concludes that individuals who are treated with respect and given autonomy by their superiors have better relations with superiors and peers and also perform better in their assigned tasks than do individuals who are closely and arbitrarily supervised. However, though it appears that supportive management styles do generate improved relations with superiors and close relations with peers, there is some evidence that such management is not consistently associated with high performance" (Wilson, 1968, p. 146).

effectuation of change, John Wax properly stresses this perspective of executive power implicit in which is the need for ethics:

> The classical sociological definition states that power is the ability to influence the beliefs and behaviors of others in accordance with a wish or plan. Another somewhat more interactional and controversial definition states that power increases as the power-holder exercises increasing influence over others, while they exercise decreasing influence over him. Two other definitions useful for our purposes are: a) Power is the control of a resource or resources which are essential to the functioning or survival of an individual or an organization. b) Power is the ability to influence behavior through the use of rewards and penalties (1971, p. 274).

The nature of the organization executive's power over organization staff does vary. It varies in relation to such variables as the size and importance of the organization; the dispensability or indispensability of the individual staff member as well as the security or insecurity of the executive; the psychological needs of the executive; the dependency of the executive on staff members; etc. But, in some degree or other, that power will exist and depend only on the executive's inclination to use, overuse, or abuse it. Moreover, whatever is real about the executive's power as far as control of resources, rewards, penalties, approval, and so on, are concerned, there is much about it that need not be real at all but require only staff members' perceptions of, and responses to it to make it work to the executive's advantage and to their disadvantage, if the executive so sees fit.

Ostensibly, staff members who belong to professions the services of which are critical to the effective functioning of social organizations—like social workers and psychologists, for example—are in a position to resist or counteract the inclination of executives to misuse their real or illusory power. And sometimes they can, as Rogers and Molnar suggest in their discussion of the possibility of conflict or ambiguity in the roles of professional staff members and executives:

> The type of services of an organization also may influence the level of conflict or ambiguity. . . . Professional roles are often permitted greater discretion and are supported by the authority of professional codes, which may conflict with organizational codes, so that there is greater possibility of conflict between the administrator and staff. . . . Multiple sources of direction tend to create uncertainty and inconsistency about organizational means and goals (1976, p. 600).

However, Rogers and Molnar go on to define autonomy as "an administrator's authority to make decisions that set the goals of the organization and determine the means for achieving them." And there is little doubt that the greater the conflict or ambiguity of roles in the organization, depending upon the executive's preferences and inclinations, the greater the executive's freedom to exercise the ultimate option. Staff members being employees—however much they may resist the designation—and executives being employers—however much they may obscure that fact—executives can, if they so choose, make the most of any existing uncertainty, with full confidence in the authority they actually do carry. All they may get in return is what has been described as "antagonistic cooperation" (Riesman, Glazer, and Denney, 1950), but what counts ultimately is what executives manage to do with what they have in the meantime.

The Ethical Responsibility of Executives to Staff

There is invariably some kind of power at the social organization executive's disposal in relation to organization staff members, which the executive is, as a matter of ethics, on one hand obliged to use in behalf of the organization and, on the other, not to misuse or abuse to the disadvantage of staff members. A few principles of ethical administrative practice may therefore be suggested as illustrative of the executive's ethical responsibility.

The beginning of the executive-staff relationship is generally the hiring process, which may be fair and considerate—which is to say ethical in the context of the ethics of social work administration—or unfair and inconsiderate. A candidate for a job, except for the indispensable expert whose interest in a job must be carefully cultivated—a rare enough exception at best—is often at the mercy of an organization executive, especially when the labor market for a particular occupation is deeply depressed.

One aspect of administrative ethics concerns the way in which the executive treats the candidate. Another is the influences which operate for the executive. The more extraneous to the executive's organizational responsibility these influences are, the less ethical the executive's actions are apt to be. An executive who likes to be surrounded by ineffectual yes-persons rather than sturdy, independent, and competent practitioners, and employs candidates on that basis, is hardly responsive to ethical responsibility to select qualified candidates for the organization, however generous the choice is to the candidates. Generosity of this kind is rarely ethical; nor is ethics a matter of generosity. Ethics does no favors. Ethics is simply a response to the obligatory:

> A "good deed" we call an action that agrees to some given standard—to an ideal of human behavior that we use as our model or to a moral imperative. . . . We cannot decide empirically on the "validity" of the value scales we use as standards. There is a relevant difference between

these standards and, for example, what one calls "standards of efficiency" which refer to a means-ends relationship. . . . In speaking of moral values . . . there is implied a direction for action, a tendency to realize those values . . . in action (Hartmann, 1960, pp. 46-49).

It is the ethical responsibility of the social organization executive to the organization—when administrative authority so permits—to select the right person for each available job and, when administrative authorization and opportunity do not so permit, to insure the thorough and judicious performance of that task by whoever does have the authority. The appointment of a personal friend may be a kindly deed to the friend who may be unemployed and in desperate need of employment, but not to the organization for which the duty of careful and suitable candidate selection is primary (cf. Garnett, 1956; and Feinberg, 1961).

It is the ethical responsibility of the executive to the candidate, on the other hand, to consider and weigh fairly the qualifications of the candidate for the available vacancy. This responsibility derives from the executive's position, and the opportunity which inheres in that position to affect the fate of a defenseless candidate. It also derives from the candidate's reliance on the executive to be treated fairly and impartially. To underscore the obvious, administrative ethics leaves no room for discrimination in the selection of staff on the basis of race, sex, religion, sexual orientation or preference, age, or any other consideration not specifically relevant to qualification for employment.

Although the executive and candidate do not yet have, and may never have an employer-employee relationship, they are parties to a functional relationship, as transitory as it may be, in which responsibility—the executive's—and risk—the candidate's—are operative.

The executive's ethical responsibility to the candidate may of course be extended when broadly-based societal values are conceded which dictate administrative responsibility—aside from that which may be legally incurred under existing legislation and governmental regulation—for preferential treatment for candidates who belong to specified groups. The issue need not be the choice of an unqualified candidate over a qualified one, but the preference for one qualified candidate of a certain physical or ethnic description over a qualified candidate of another description. This insures that the responsibility to the organization is not overlooked. The problem is to avoid unethical consequences for others.

The issue to be contended with is the relative fairness of the final choice of candidate. Since values are in effect arbitrary, though in this case based on a variety of considerations related to and affecting the administrative situation encountered, what will be regarded as ethical will be that choice most compatible with the value to which priority is assigned.

Exploiting an Applicant's Vulnerabilities

One of the more bitter uses of executive power is the exploitation by an executive of the vulnerability of a job applicant who is obviously desperate for a job. The offense to ethics is not only that such a candidate may not be hired or may be hired cheaply, but also interviewed and considered in a degrading and demeaning manner. Although it is a truism that one generally does better to seek employment while employed, ethics requires of executives the same high order of treatment whether the applicant is already employed or not. The ethics of social work administration would make imperative the considerate and fair treatment of candidates for employment no matter how low their status or how high their vulnerability, and perhaps all the more so precisely because of either. Ethical responsibility implies that what the party at risk in an occupational relationship cannot provide for himself or herself, it is incumbent upon the party with the power in that relationship—the party with the occupational responsibility in it at any rate—to provide.

Exploiting Staff Vulnerabilities

If the dependency of prospective candidates is a significant consideration in defining the ethical responsibility of executives to them, it is hardly less a consideration in defining the ethical responsibility of executives to staff members who depend on them to retain the jobs they already have (cf. Emerson, 1962), a consideration characteristic of employer-employee relationships in social organizations (cf. Mills, 1956, p. 224). Work, being "the central fact of our lives" (Dubin, 1958, p. 3), this dependency of staff members, whatever its intensity, and the ethical responsibility of executives which is associated with it, loom large in the relationship between executive and staff.

Functional Relevance of Executive Expectations

At its most primitive, an executive's offense in this connection may take the form of sexual advances toward a staff member, or even setting as a precondition for keeping a job, if not getting the job in the first place, ready access to sexual favors. But it is sufficient to the purposes of administrative ethics for an executive to talk or gesture in terms of the gender of an employee when not relevant to the employee's organizational function or role. A pinch on an employee's rear end, for example, may not only be as offensive to the employee as a "pass," or any other lewd and lascivious gesture or suggestion, but also as unethical as far as principles of ethical administrative practice are concerned. In this context, it is as inappropriate to talk about degrees of unethical conduct as it is to talk about degrees of pregnancy. Obviously some offenses are more consequential than others, particularly in relation to a staff member's relatively disadvantaged position as compared with an executive, and particularly in relation to the risks for the staff member because of that position.

More subtle, though not less insidious, are those actions taken by executives in relation to staff members, or those demands made by executives of staff members, in exclusive reliance upon the authority of the executives. Such actions and demands must be regarded as unethical when they have no bearing on their necessity or utility for valid organizational purposes, or their appropriateness in relation to staff members' organizational functions. It is only an incrementally greater offense for executives to demand of administratively intimidated staff members unethical, compromising, insulting, illegal, or organizationally dysfunctional actions.

It is bad enough—ethically speaking—for executives to "pull rank" arbitrarily and without regard to the organizational purposes for which administrative rank is primarily designed. It is worse for executives, in doing so, to subvert the purposes to which the organization is institutionally committed, or the means by which those purposes may be effectively served. This, in itself, is a betrayal of administrative duty. It is a major violation to commit these offenses to ethics and to premise them on the expectation or necessity of unethical conduct on the part of staff members.

Codes of professional ethics usually provide for the encouragement of ethical conduct on the part of colleagues in general. It would be an *a fortiori* expectation of practitioners that they do not require unethical conduct of colleagues, particularly when they have the weight of administrative authority behind them. The NASW Code of Ethics, for example, not only *pro*scribes the taking or inducing of unethical actions; it also *pre*scribes principles which emphasize the affirmative responsibility of social workers—all social workers, not simply administrators—to encourage others to be ethical, and to discourage and even prevent the unethical conduct of others. These principles also admonish social workers to take action against those who do engage in unethical conduct. The way these principles are phrased makes quite evident their applicability to social organization executives:

> The social worker should create and maintain conditions of practice that facilitate ethical and competent performance by colleagues. . . . The social worker should take action through appropriate channels against unethical conduct by any other member of the profession (1979).

The role of the social organization executive in inspiring, inducing, and facilitating ethical conduct on the part of organization staff members in all of their occupational relationships and transactions is obviously an important one. For the executive to engage in unethical conduct or to require it of others is hardly responsive to the expectations of that role.

Naturally, judgment is called for in determining what is and what is not ethical, and what the proper choice of action is when a number of actions appear to be obligatory but not all can be taken. However, guides are available in occupational codes and commentaries.

Most difficult, though hardly impossible, is the employment of occupational discretion when a choice must be made between ethical responsibility to staff and ethical responsibility to others or to the social organization. For this purpose, systematic though often rapid analysis is necessary of all of the applicable ethical responsibilities and all of the available options, including those to which and to whom priority may be owed, and under what circumstances.

The duty of the social organization executive is of course complex in this regard. The duty to organization staff members is itself complex enough, but nevertheless generally clear, particularly in light of the relatively disadvantaged position of staff members as compared with the executive, and in light of the executive's defined authority and responsibility in relation to staff.

Power, unfortunately, often grows by what it feeds on. "He who has acquired power will almost always endeavor to consolidate it and to extend it, to multiply the ramparts which defend his position" (Michels, 1966, p. 206). Executives—some more so than others—are not always above consolidating their positions and making maximum use of them. What is more, they are not always above resorting to one layer of influence over staff members in order to reinforce another, at times to advance their own self-interest whether sexual, organizational, or vocational. The threat of a blacklist or a negative reference may be held over the head of a recalcitrant or uncooperative staff member, if the threat of unemployment will not do the trick. The threat may not even have to be made if the staff member suspects the possibility of its implementation—as unrealistic as that perception may prove to be.

Evaluation, References, and Dismissal

It would not only be a lie about a staff member's performance that would be unethical. It is also the misuse of the truth that is unethical—in the form of an actual or implied threat, for example. Again, the reason that it is unethical, fundamentally, is that this is not what evaluations and references are for. This is not their function. This is not what executives are—to cast things in a value framework—supposed to do with them. It is unethical for executives to use them to obscure the truth or to serve any purpose other than that for which they are designed—both internally for the organization, and externally in relation to future employers.

The truth includes the critical truth. As Virginia Robinson put it in relation to student social work supervision, "to refrain from criticism at points where there is a definite standard on which to base it, is not kindness" (1936, p. 101). As between executives and staff members, evaluative statements made in references, written evaluations, or in personal conferences, to be ethical, should include such criticism as may be validated. It is of course more humane to use such criticism constructively, but as an ethical requisite this may have to be placed in the realm of greater ambiguity. On the other hand, there is nothing especially ethical about wielding criticism like a sledge hammer, and deriving gratification by seeing a criticized staff member squirm in a chair.

Before dismissal of a staff member is considered, on the basis of validated evidence of serious deficiency or incompetence, opportunities for staff growth and improvement ought, as a matter of ethical responsibility, to be exhausted. Upon demonstrable evidence of failure in all attempts to effect change in the staff member to accord with reasonable expectations in job performance, the process of dismissal is then maximally considerate and humane, with maximum consideration for the dignity and future opportunities of the staff member. The executive remains ethically responsible to perform the necessary administrative functions which affect staff members, but not without conscientious fulfillment of ethical responsibility toward them. Prior to dismissal, however, great care and consideration are ethically required in the process of staff development and evaluation. Similar care and consideration are required in the preparation of reference letters about staff members.

Administrative Ethics and the Developmental Needs of Staff

One view of administrative ethics, as I have implied, expands considerably the ethical responsibility of administrators to include the maximization of effort in the interest of the personal development and advancement of organization staff members (cf., for example, Levy, 1973, p. 20). It is hardly excessive to expect executives to make possible, if not likely, the successful performance by staff members of their assigned organization functions by providing an adequate orientation to those functions, and by insuring the means necessary for performing them. Helpful guidance for staff members toward the performance of their assigned functions represents an important component of administrative ethics.

Social organization executives can, should they be of a mind to do so, perpetrate their unethical conduct by what may appear to an observer to be indirection. This makes such an outcome no less unethical since ethics may be reflected in "acts" of omission as well as commission. In fact, a favored technique of some executives is to let subordinates do what the executives themselves are responsible to do and, with a bit of effort, could do. This is a treatment of choice for executives who prefer to keep their own hands "clean." Executives sometimes employ "hatchet men" (or women) to do the "dirty work" they would rather not be associated with—either out of frank cowardice, or the pretense of saintliness. The "dirty work" is usually that of firing staff members without real cause or making them sufficiently miserable to resign. The true "cause" may be the executive's convenience because the staff member raises too many questions, or displeases a board member who then puts pressure on the executive to do something about it. Or the cause may be economic—a new, young staff member may cost less than an older, more highly paid one.

Unsettling Staff: The Politics of Administration

Another technique with which executives circumvent their ethical responsibility to organization staff members is to drop disquieting hints—usually via unofficial emissaries—that the collective functioning of staff members is not in all respects measuring up to standard. This technique is invidiously enhanced by being studiously vague about what it is that is being done that is so faulty, and about the standard that is being applied—with no better purpose to be served than to unsettle the staff, a kind of one-upmanship by one-downing. It takes less than that to unsettle staff members who are not confident about their standing to begin with—this being another reflection of questionable and unethical administrative practice. As neither objective nor as instrumentality can such a device, however passive, be regarded as ethical, violating as it does any number of the conventions of conduct in relation to organization colleagues. It has particular significance in relation to subordinates, since they do not enjoy equal protection with the executive.

Another, perhaps more complex technique sometimes employed by executives is, in its fundamentals, a rather old one. It both resorts to, and generates, intraorganizational competition and rivalry, and the exploitation of administrative biases and preferences. Both its means and its ends are unethical on their face. It is the sort of technique that exploits what Pfeffer and Salancik describe as a political process in organizational decision-making (1974). They are talking about university budgets, but the findings of their study apply to social organizations and their processes in general, especially large organizations.

> Organizational decision-making and particularly resource allocation decision-making is a political process and can be explained by consideration of relative subunit power, as well as by consideration of possible bureaucratic criteria. . . . To the extent a subunit has power within the organization the department has an advantage in obtaining resources regardless of the work load (pp. 139, 148).

Pfeffer and Salancik also assert that "Political power, in addition to being used to obtain organizational resources, may be used more subtly to obtain the use of universalistic criteria that happen to favor one sub-unit's position" (p. 136). These become considerations for the ethics of social work administration in that executives, out of fairness to organizational sub-units in budgeting, allocations, and assignments, are obliged to make sure that it is not political power and political acumen that determine what is decided and what is done. Executives are certainly obliged not to exploit the existing power of sub-units to attain ends that they happen to prefer.

Similar responsibility accrues to executives in relation to coordination, which can be used either to serve constructive organizational purposes fairly and justly, or to obstruct them and to misuse staff. Intraorganizationally, coordination becomes especially urgent when interdependence and conflict among an organization's sub-units are especially great (cf. Pondy, 1970). The avoidance of internecine strife, on one hand, and the attainment of cooperative effort, on the other, as well as the effectuation of equity among staff sub-units and among staff members, are administrative responsibilities which are required for effective coordination. They are also ethical responsibilities for organization executives. They are affirmative in that they are designed for the implementation of the important administrative function of coordination that it is the duty of executives to perform. These responsibilities also have negative connotations in that executives are duty-bound not to exploit staff interdependence and conflict to satisfy personal preferences. Executives are also duty-bound not to passively permit interdependence and conflict to run their own destructive course without intervention.

The Ethics of Personnel Practices

Mary Hester's brief for a specific, complete, and clearly written statement of personnel practices is, in effect, a summary of the ethical responsibility of executives to organization staff members. Such a statement, she says,

> is essential in establishing and maintaining good executive-staff relationships. . . . The value of such a statement, of course, is in the security felt by staff in recognized and agreed upon rights, duties, and conditions of work as well as expectations concerning salary and promotions, which are the same for all and are not subject to arbitrary and hastily made conditions and decisions. Staff members then are not in the position of asking or having "favors" granted; they know where they stand. . . . There should be genuine respect for differing points of view and the staff should be accepted as a responsible partner . . . machinery should be provided to insure the staff member an impartial review of the executive's decision when he feels an injustice has been done (1946, pp. 44, 46).

Such measures are obviously compatible with the ethics of social work administration, although a personnel practices code of the kind Hester describes is also an administrative document. The former emphasizes the value-based expectations of administrative practice, including personnel practices. The latter emphasizes the practical substance of personnel practices. Whether or not such provisions are recorded in such a document, or provided for in a union contract, it is the ethical responsibility of the social organization executive to live by them. They may not even be sufficient, in fact, for administrative ethics extends beyond the call of legislated duty.

A code of ethics governing the relationship of the social organization executive and the organization staff would no doubt be an extensive one, but, like occupational codes in general, even that might not be sufficient:

> The inherent limitation in ethical codes is the leeway they leave for human judgment and for balancing competing values. Without such leeway, any code would be unworkable; with it, the code is open to evasion. Application of ethical principles to real cases is literally a problem in casuistry and is vulnerable to the abuses that give casuistry a bad name. . . . Insofar as there is no objective, common measure by which competing values can be "traded off," the fallibility of human judgment cannot be eliminated from decisions (Smith, 1967, p. 56).

Codes of ethics can indeed do only so much. Well-constructed, however, they do afford guidance for the exercise of the kind of discretion that executives are inevitably called upon to exercise in resolving issues of ethics that arise in relation to staff members. In the meantime—that is, until such a code is made available—executives must seek guidance where they can find it. This includes codes which do exist and which are relevant to their assignments and functions, or by which they are governed as members of particular occupations. Such norms as apply to their organizations, or the fields of practice and endeavor with which their organizations are associated—like child welfare and rehabilitation—also afford guidance. But, in the last analysis, executives must act as their own guides. When they do so act, they act not on the basis of their own private and personal values, preferences, and predilections, but on the basis of values and expectations derived from several specific sources. These include their administrative responsibility; the power it induces for them; and the effects and implications both have for others to whom they therefore have ethical responsibility. For such responsibility, executives must feel an ultimate accountability. Among those to whom social organization executives have ethical responsibility, organization staff members are especially prominent.

REFERENCES

Alutto, Joseph A. and Acito, Franklin. "Decisional Participation and Sources of Job Satisfaction: A Study of Manufacturing Personnel," Working Paper Series 160 (State University of New York at Buffalo, School of Management) N.D., c. 1970. Mimeographed.

Alutto, Joseph A. and Belasco, James A. "A Typology for Participation in Organizational Decision-Making," *Administrative Science Quarterly,* 17 (1972), 117-125.

Argyris, Chris. "Personality and Organization Theory Revisited," *Administrative Science Quarterly,* 18 (1973a), 141-167.

Argyris, Chris. "Some Limits of Rational Man Organization Theory," *Public Administration Review,* 33 (1973b), 253-267.

Berliner, Arthur K. "Some Pitfalls in Administrative Behavior," *Social Casework,* 52 (1971), 562-566.

Carlton, Thomas Owen. "Improving Management in Social Welfare Agencies Through Increased Participation," *Journal of Social Welfare,* 3 (1976), 45-56.

Cusson, Maurice and Laberge-Altmejd, Danielle. "L'Exercise Du Pouvoir En Institution," *Crime and/et Justice,* 4 (1977), 238-254.

Dubin, Robert. *The World of Work: Industrial Society and Human Relations* (Englewood Cliffs, N.J.: Prentice-Hall, 1958).

Emerson, Richard M. "Power-Dependence Relations," *American Sociological Review,* 27 (1962), 31-41.

Etzioni, Amitai. *A Comparative Analysis of Complex Organizations: On Power, Involvements, and Their Correlates* (Revised and Enlarged Ed.; New York: The Free Press, 1975).

Etzioni, Amitai. "A Creative Adaptation to a World of Rising Shortages," *The Annals of the American Academy of Political and Social Science* 420 (1975), 98-110.

Feinberg, Joel. "Supererogation and Rules," *Ethics,* 71 (1961), 276-288.

Garnett, A. Campbell. "The Indicative Element in Deontological Words," *Ethics,* 67 (1956), 42-52.

Hartmann, Heinz. *Psychoanalysis and Moral Values* (New York: International Press, 1960).

Hester, Mary. "The Executive and the Staff," in Helen W. Hanchette *et al., Some Dynamics of Social Agency Administration* (New York: Family Service Association of America, 1946), 36-54.

Levy, Charles S. "The Ethics of Supervision," *Social Work,* 18 (1973), 14-21.

Michels, Robert. *Political Parties.* Trans. Eden and Cedar Paul (New York: The Free Press, 1966).

Mills, C. Wright. *White Collar* (New York: Oxford University Press, 1956).

National Association of Social Workers. Code of Ethics, Adopted by NASW Delegate Assembly, November 18, 1979 (see Appendix).

Pfeffer, Jeffrey and Salancik, Gerald R. "Organizational Decision-Making as a Political Process: The Case of the University Budget," *Administrative Science Quarterly,* 19 (1974), 135-151.

Pfiffner, John M. and Sherwood, Frank P. *Administrative Organization* (Englewood Cliffs, N.J.: Prentice-Hall, 1960).

Pondy, Louis R. "Interdependence, Conflict, and Coordination in Organizations," GSBA Paper No. 32, revised version, October, 1970 (Graduate School of Business Administration, Duke University) Mimeographed.

Presthus, Robert. *The Organizational Society: An Analysis and a Theory* (New York: Vintage Books, 1962).

Riesman, David with Glazer, Nathan and Denney, Reuel. *The Lonely Crowd: A Study of the Changing American Character* (New Haven: Yale University Press, 1950).

Robinson, Virginia P. *Supervision in Social Case Work* (Chapel Hill, N.C.: The University of North Carolina Press, 1936).

Rogers, David L. and Molnar, Joseph. "Organizational Antecedents of Role Conflict and Ambiguity in Top-Level Administrators," *Administrative Science Quarterly,* 21 (1976), 598-610.

Scott, William G. "Organization Government: The Prospects for a Truly Participative System," *Public Administration Review,* 29 (1969), 43-52.

Smith, M. Brewster. "Conflicting Values Affecting Behavioral Research with Children," *Children,* 14 (1967), 53-58.

Trecker, Harleigh B. *Group Process in Administration* (Revised and Enlarged Ed.; New York: Woman's Press, 1950).

Wax, John, "Power Theory and Institutional Change," *The Social Service Review,* 45 (1971), 274-288.

Wilson, Thomas P. "Patterns of Management and Adaptations to Organizational Roles: A Study of Prison Inmates," *The American Journal of Sociology,* 74 (1968), 146-157.

IX. THE EXECUTIVE AND THE WORLD OUTSIDE THE ORGANIZATION

I have suggested that executives of social organizations may be the least autonomous of practitioners in human service organizations. Whatever the organization is accountable for, its executive is answerable for.

> The agency is accountable 1) to its members or participants, 2) to its directors or trustees, 3) to the community chest which gives financial aid, and ultimately 4) to the community. The agency must answer not only for its use of funds but also must produce evidence of its usefulness, because the success of a charitable organization is measured not in dollars but in the services rendered the community. Nevertheless, unless financial facts are carefully recorded and interpreted the institution will not survive, because it will not be able to instill confidence in the public mind and sustain good will (Youngwood, 1949, p. 3).

Administrative Ethics in the Interorganizational and Community Spheres

The answerability of the social organization executive, however, is not based upon its practical necessity alone. The failure of the executive to give a sufficient accounting of the organization's services and programs or of its finances may, of course, have negative consequences for the organization. However, the problem for the executive is not merely the risk of losing the public's confidence and good will. The problem which merits the executive's concern from an ethical point of view is also that the public's confidence and good will must be merited. The administrative responsibility to make the accounting to the community is also ethical responsibility therefore.

From the point of view of the ethics of social work administration, executives are not free to do as they please either in the organization or outside of it. The ethics of social work administration applies as much to the world around the social organization as the world within it. To a great extent, the ethics of social work administration in relation to the world around the social organization depends more upon the initiative and good offices of the organization's executive than that in the organization. One of the reasons for this is that the interests of the organization as an organization—as distinguished from the social functions for which the organization is accountable—sometimes conflict with the executive's ethical responsibility to others outside the organization.

Occasionally, the better part of administrative ethics is precisely the preservation for the organization of its own autonomy. For example, governmental funding of voluntary agencies often represents a threat to organizational autonomy. It is perfectly reasonable to expect the organization's executive to abide by the policies of the funding agency, and to be responsive to the organization's moral obligations to that agency. It would be unethical of the executive not to. On the other hand, the executive also owes to the organization such cautions and such efforts as militate against the selling of its institutional soul for a mess of porridge, particularly if the conditions of the funding in any way contradict or subvert the organization's avowed purposes and intentions. The line between the two types of ethical responsibility can be mighty thin sometimes[1] (cf. Kramer, 1979, pp. 7-12).

Similarly, relationships with other social organizations are often necessary for the coordination of services and for continuity of care for clienteles. But

> such linkages are not necessarily constructive, however. Under certain circumstances they can have problematic consequences for organizations and their personnel . . . Cooperation among agencies may take the form of bargaining, cooptation, or coalition. Each of these modes of relating diminishes the organization's autonomy. . . . Moreover, each exacts increasing costs in terms of the staff's time and effort (Wilson, 1978, pp. 14,17).[2]

In each of these cases, the value by which social organization executives are expected to be guided as a matter of administrative ethics in relation to the world outside the organization—to other public or voluntary organizations in these cases—is that of cooperation, colored by accountability. But ethics also requires of organization executives the anticipation and consideration of organization and perhaps service cost. The very consideration of both is a function of the executive's ethical responsibility. The outcome should be the result of a weighing and weighting of ethical priorities for a determination of which of the executive's moral obligations merits priority and what approach to its fulfillment is clearly ethical. For the ethics of instrumentalities deserves as much attention as the ethics of their intended outcomes.

---

[1]"Organizational and communal ends sometimes conflict with service and relational obligations and not infrequently . . . the former are accorded disproportionately more priority than the latter. . . . Religion can be one provocation. Vested interests can be another. And misguided judgment can be still another" (Levy, 1977, p. 21).

[2]"The network of organizations . . . consists of a number of distinguishable organizations having a significant amount of interaction with each other. Such interaction may at one extreme include extensive, reciprocal exchanges of resources or intense hostility and conflict at the other. . . . Considerations of resource adequacy determine, within fairly restrictive limits, the nature of interactions in the performance of mandated functions" (Benson, 1975, pp. 230-231).

Autonomy: Executive's or Organization's

The autonomy to which executives are obliged to accord priority in relation to extra-organizational demands is not theirs but that of the organizations. It is not the will of the executives that is at stake, but the institutional options of their employing organizations. The will of the executives might be a valid consideration were the issue for them the impartial and independent exercise of occupational discretion. This implies full, objective, and unintimidated use of their occupational knowledge and skill, and scrupulous application of principles of ethical practice to their administrative and organizational as well as social responsibility.

Whether executives are moved by organizational considerations or subjective considerations, their zeal for freedom of movement is often evoked by the hazards they perceive—not always unrealistically—in their and their organizations' relationship to other organizations and the community at large. The result is sometimes unethical conduct, or at least the neglect of ethical responsibility in the interorganizational sphere—in the relationship between social organizations and other organizations:

> The political economy theory is closely related to the resource control theory of organizational effectiveness proposed by Yuchtman and Seashore. This theory states that critically needed resources are in short supply in the environment and consequently the ability of an organization to survive and prosper is a function of its ability to *outmaneuver* other organizations in the acquisition of these scarce resources. An effective organization, therefore, is characterized as having a strong *bargaining* position which enables it to *dominate* its environment. . . . Yuchtman and Seashore, and others have pointed out that administrators are accountable to multiple constituencies which utilize conflicting criteria for measuring organizational effectiveness (Whetten, 1978, p. 255; emphasis supplied).

The underscored words connote unethical conduct in the interorganizational sphere in that they describe opportunistic rather than cooperative behavior, designed more in organizational self-interest than in collective social, communal, and consumer interest. The focus is on who can get there first and get out with the most, rather than—as ethical responsibility to clients, community, and society would dictate—what must be done with available resources in order to serve clients better and most economically; and in order to do what must be done, and done best, and by whom for the well-being of the community.

Acting for their organizations, executives can go to great lengths in vying with other organizations for a disproportionate share of available resources— disproportionate at least in relation to existing needs and in relation to the relative capacity of their own organizations to meet those needs as compared with the capacity of other organizations.[3]

The Executive and Extra-Organizational Colleagues: Fair and Unfair Competition

Principles of ethical practice are needed to guide the conduct of executives in their dealings with colleagues in other organizations with which they must compete for limited resources. They are duty-bound to represent well the interests of their own organizations, but their actions in the fulfillment of their duty, to be ethical, must at the same time be contained within the boundaries of inter-collegial decency and fairness. For example,

> Ethical principles might be identified which could help Jewish organizations avoid the destructive impact of acts perpetrated in predatory competition and strife with other Jewish organizations—acts which sometimes do occur in the organizational struggle for community resources and approval, or institutional self-preservation and aggrandizement (Levy, 1977, p. 21).

Social organization executives are under constant pressure—especially when their organizations are under pressure—either to prove the validity of their organizations as organizations, or to outdistance other organizations in the quest for funds, approval, or plain attention. The loyalty of executives to their organizations is constantly being tested, with expectations sometimes reaching unseemly extremes as far as administrative ethics is concerned, especially in relation to outside organizations and persons. Executives may, in fact, be expected—by organization boards, for example—to adhere to a double standard of administrative conduct: rigidly pure inside the organization and somewhat tainted outside the organization. Accountability may mean one thing for the board in the organization, and something else outside the organization. Not that the board is a collection of thieves; only that standards may be a little more elastic for one set of purposes than for another—as in the use of government funds as compared with board-raised funds. The interpretation of accountability is apt to differ, for example. A generally acceptable view may be something like the following:

---

[3]"In the examination of resource allocations to member agencies within United Funds, we have found . . . empirical support for the power-dependence framework which has been proposed to explain interorganizational relations. . . . As predicted, power was related to the dependence relationship existing between the agency and the United Fund and was a function of both the agency's ability to attract outside resources and the importance of the agency to the Fund. . . . The contest for resources plays an important part in determining organizational and interorganizational behavior" (Pfeffer and Leong, 1977, p. 788).

The key word in traditional budgeting is "accountability," and the essence of the orientation is "control: i.e., how do you prevent public funds from being stolen, used for unauthorized purposes or spent at uncontrolled rates. . . . The task of those who approve the budget is to economize by acquiring inputs at the lowest cost and to "keep the lid" on total costs (Galnoor and Gross, 1969, p. 25).

But, as Galnoor and Gross go on to demonstrate, the process of the accounting may prove time-, manpower-, and resource-consuming and still produce only useless and unused results (p. 42). And yet, the organization's leaders, including the executive, may rest content as long the requirements are met, however superficially, and as long as the organization's fiscal ends continue to be attained.

On the other hand, organization leaders may act like a bunch of skinflints in allocating and spending money on staff and services and, at the same time, luxuriate at parties and meetings, with twelve-year old scotch whiskey and finely honed hors d'oeuvres, all at organization expense, without a twinge of conscience.

Social organization executives have their occupational consciences and a tight ethical wire to traverse. They are required to choose, from moment to moment, conduct which is responsive to their organizational responsibility and yet ethical in relation to others outside the organization; and conduct which is responsive to the dictates and conventions of inter-collegial and interorganizational courtesy and fair play, and yet loyal to their organizations. Sometimes, of course, the choice is not to be ethical to one or the other. In that case, compelling considerations which can be documented ought to be offered in justification of the deviation for, in the context of the ethics of social work administration, that is what it is.

Subjective Intrusions on Administrative Ethics

A more seductive distraction for the ethics of social organization executives occurs when they are beset by personal needs and aspirations which make ethical choices of administrative action a strain for them. The urge to succeed, or the fear of failure; or the desire simply to *look* successful at all costs, whatever the truth of the matter may be, induces behavior which may not always, or in all respects, be ethical. Executives, under such circumstances, prefer to be exempt from accountability, to do what they feel impelled to do, without regard to what is owed by way of ethical responsibility to others. Under such circumstances, the competition of executives for funds, for example, may be vicious, and presentations for allocations may skirt the truth. Or the power at their disposal may be overused or misused without regard for what might otherwise be a more equitable distribution of resources. Similarly erratic or excessive conduct may apply to other spheres of administrative practice.

In the realm of resource allocation, as in other realms of administrative practice, it is not necessary for executives to feel a particular compulsion to succeed in order to ply their advantage over colleagues in other organizations. All they need feel is the comfort and the temptations of their advantage—as long as they get "theirs"! Whether it is in their organizations' interest or their own for executives to have this view, it neglects the broader view and the broader vision which is an essential part of the ethics of social work administration. The broader view includes a concern about what is the best for the most, and what is most needed in the community.

The Ethics of Organizational Evaluation

The social organization executive is morally obligated to examine or to have examined, honestly and candidly, every aspect of the organization's purposes and practices, without permitting personal aspirations and biases to distort or obscure the process or the results. Such an examination represents the organization's accounting to the community for the organization's efforts and their outcomes. The ethics of social work administration requires an accurate accounting even if the risk is reduced allocations and support. Again, of course, this kind of ethical system does not work well in parts. It does not work if some "do" and some "do not." When this happens the inequity falls to the conscientious executive and organization. Equity in this connection is hard to come by. As Aaron Rosenblatt has suggested:

> The evaluator of a service program is often subject to serious economic, political, or social pressures. This is especially so when the results of a study have important, immediate consequences for board members, administrators, staff members, or recipients of service. . . . Ideology, politics, or personal gain can distort the interpretation of results. . . . Those who control the purse strings have a more than academic interest in the results.
>
> Administrators and staff members also show a keen interest . . . In extreme cases their jobs may be at stake (1977, p. 93).

This statement recalls for me an evaluation conference I once conducted as an agency administrator, in which was discussed the issue of the use of part-time staff for supervisory field functions. When the implication began to emerge that the agency's service purposes might be better served by the employment of full-time staff in lieu of part-time staff, one of the part-time staff members indignantly asserted that he would be damned if he was going to participate in, and contribute data to a discussion a consequence of which might be his own dismissal. Well, he was honest about it. It takes a person of rather large qualitative stature to serve the truth at his or her expense, and yet that is precisely what the ethics of social work administration demands.

Perhaps this helps to explain what Johnson and Taylor discovered to represent the "planning contradiction" in social agencies, planning being, in effect, the obverse side of organizational evaluation. Executives might appear to favor the kind of planning upon which evaluation is properly based, or which is properly based on evaluation, and yet settle for a low or nonexistent level of planning in their organizations.

> Indeed, *absence* of extensive planning may allow some administrators to reduce conflict within their agencies and to preserve personal prerogatives and authority. Planning activity may be perceived as running the risk that conflicting points of view will be aired and that groups not normally participating in the administrative process will become active in the examination of policies and programs. Planning, in short, may be perceived by some administrators as a vehicle for the introduction of uncertainty and risk. . . . If social services are public commodities that, at least in part, "belong" to existing and potential consumers of service, then executives who do not utilize systematic and institutionalized planning mechanisms are denying important segments of the community an opportunity to participate in scanning alternatives before final decisions are made (Johnson and Taylor, 1978, pp. 179-180).

Johnson and Taylor put very well here one of the major premises of administrative ethics in relation to the world outside the social organization, for they emphasize the responsibility of executives to others outside the organization. That premise is the relationship and responsibility of the executive to others, each being a consequence of the other and a reason for the other. Whether the executive carries out the responsibility, and the way in which it is done, if indeed it is done, matters to others, not only inside the organization but outside as well. The ethics of social work administration is thus not only an intramural dynamic. It stretches far beyond the organization's walls to other social organizations, the community, and society.[4] Evaluation is one of its manifestations.

What makes the ethics of social work administration especially unwieldy is

---

[4]Brouillette and Quarantelli identify internal organizational factors and external factors which affect the way in which organizations adapt to large-scale stress. The internal factors include perceived demands, nature of the bureaucratic structure, emergency capability, and perceived effectiveness and efficiency. The external factors which influence the adaptive responses of organizations include situational factors, the space-time or ecological dimension, interorganizational relationships in the community under stress, and the community and societal contexts (1971). All of these factors operate for the social organization executive. In addition, the executive is moved by even less rational stimuli and entirely subjective inclinations and self-interest. How much of the latter depends a great deal on the executive's administrative and ethical discipline and constraint.

its relative unamenability to objective analysis and appraisal. As George and Wilding insist about views on the welfare state, the ethics of social work administration represents "a fusion of scientific evidence and of ideology" (1976, p. 22). As they suggest about fundamental issues of welfare provision in general, "ideology plays a more important part than scientific evidence" in contentions with issues in administrative ethics, "for on such issues there can be little true evidence."

But the ethics of social work administration is not entirely unamenable to systematic and rational analysis even if it is based on values. Ethics does have its logic. Ethics does have its premises. It is up to the social organization executive to consider both in making administrative decisions and taking administrative actions.

REFERENCES

Benson, J. Kenneth. "The Interorganizational Network as a Political Economy," *Administrative Science Quarterly,* 20 (1975), 229-249.

Brouillette, John R. and Quarantelli, E. L. "Types of Patterned Variation in Bureaucratic Adaptations to Organizational Stress," *Sociological Inquiry,* 41 (1971), 39-46.

Galnoor, Itzhak and Gross, Betram M. "The New Systems Budgeting and the Developing Nations," *International Social Science Journal,* 21 (1969), 23-44.

George, Vic and Wilding, Paul. *Ideology and Social Welfare* (London: Routledge and Kegan Paul, 1976).

Johnson, Bruce S. and Taylor, Samuel H. "The Planning Contradiction in Social Agencies: Great Expectations Versus Satisfaction with Limited Performance," *Administration in Social Work,* 2 (1978), 171-181.

Kramer, Ralph M. "Public Fiscal Policy and Voluntary Agencies in Welfare States," *Social Service Review,* 53 (1979), 1-14.

Levy, Charles S. "A Code of Ethics for Jewish Communal Service?" *Journal of Jewish Communal Service,* 54 (1977), 18-25.

Pfeffer, Jeffrey and Leong, Anthony. "Resource Allocations in United Funds: Examination of Power and Dependence," *Social Forces,* 53 (1977), 775-790.

Rosenblatt, Aaron. "Integrating Null Findings of Evaluative Studies," *Journal of Social Service Research,* 1 (1977), 39-104.

Whetten, David A. "Coping with Incompatible Expectations: An Integrated View of Role Conflict," *Administrative Science Quarterly,* 23 (1978), 254-271.

Wilson, Paul. "Linkages Among Organizations: Considerations and Consequences," *Health and Social Work,* 3 (1978), 14-33.

Youngwood, Milton, "Accounting for Social Agencies," *The New York Certified Public Accountant,* 19 (1949), 3-15.

X. ON BEING AND BECOMING
AN ETHICAL EXECUTIVE

It is often difficult to be ethical. It is not surprising, therefore, that the challenge to social organization executives in deciding upon an ethical course of administrative action is so often a great one. The choice to be made by an executive in relation to an issue of ethics, when extreme conflict is experienced, is usually that between conduct preferred on the basis of occupational values—values which generate the executive's moral obligations to whoever is involved in or affected by the issue—and conduct conducive to the comfort, security, success, advancement, etc., of the executive.

The Inconvenience of Administrative Ethics

To put this another way, the reason it is often difficult for an executive to be ethical is that there are always so many "good" reasons not to be ethical— "good" of course meaning practical in relation to the self-interests or convenience of either the executive or the social organization as a whole. I include convenience because ethics can be a bloody nuisance sometimes. It is a nuisance to have to account to anyone else, or to account for obligations to anyone else. It is a nuisance to engage in an extensive process of negotiation or consideration in order to insure provision for the rights, privileges, and vulnerabilities of others, or for moral obligations owed to them. It ties an executive's tongue and hands to avoid the risks to others which are a consequence of the executive's responsibilities to them, and their reliance upon the executive to fulfill them.

The Need for Administrative Ethics

The risks and hazards for others in executives' choices of action, or their failure to act, include the omission of obligatory interventions—the failure of executives to do what they have been assigned to do, or what may be implicit in what they have been assigned to do. This leaves undone or unattended what others need or have the right to have done. The risks and hazards include also the manner in which executives do or neglect to do what is expected of them in the line of administrative duty. Either may be disadvantageous to others to-whom executives have responsibility. Either may deprive them of the respect, the dignity, the options and all of the other assets and privileges to which they might otherwise have access were they not locked into a direct or indirect relationship with the executives or dependent upon them for the performance of their administrative functions.

For some who may be affected by what social organization executives do or fail to do—like their employing organizations, for example, or clients, members and staff—the risk may take the form of neglected or improperly executed and administered services, programs and personnel policies. For them and for others the risk may take the form of ineptly designed or implemented procedures presumed to facilitate and expedite the performance of organization functions, and account for them. For still others—like community organizations, funding institutions, and contributors, for example—the risk may take the form of improper or unauthorized use of funds and other resources, or questionable means for acquiring or accounting for them.[1] The deeds, the omissions, and the misdeeds of social organization executives are therefore the "business" of many other persons and institutions.

Ethics as Time-Consuming

The ethics of social work administration is also time-consuming—more so in many ways than that of business and industrial organizations, for example. The objective in social organizations is not, as it is in these other organizations, primarily to do what needs to be done as well and as economically—and for some, as profitably—as possible. These may be influential considerations for social organizations also, but not indispensable ones, not at least at the expense of humaneness, honesty, and fairness. Just as the efficiency of the means of social organizations, and the effectiveness of their outcomes, are subject to external as well as internal appraisal, the values which guide both are subject to critical review. More than that, their administrative practices and procedures, and the relationship of the practices and procedures to their services and programs are subject to ethical screening. That, at least, is the societal expectation, an expectation rooted in the social purposes of social organizations, and the sanction they are accorded by government or community to perform their functions. Social organization executives are the duly appointed monitors of the manifest values and ethics of social organizations, and the symbolic representations of them in and outside of the organizations.

The Pervasiveness of Ethics in Social Work Administration

Social organization executives are implicitly charged to perform their administrative functions, and to see to the performance of the functions of others, with maximum fairness and considerateness, and maximum accountability, to

---

[1] A fairly extensive range of responsibilities affecting the manner in which funds are raised and accounted for by social organizations is outlined in Levy, 1973, pp. 20-32.

all who serve, and are served and affected by social organizations. They are similarly accountable to all who contribute to the organizations, and to all in whose behalf they are presumed to function, and for whom they represent a sacred trust. The position of social organizations, and therefore of their executives, is analogous to that of property-holders in some religions—they do not own the property: they simply are trustees for that property, ownership being lodged in a Supreme Being. For executives, however, the stakes are not mere property. Not only the actions but the very being of executives is affected. The weight of their responsibility can thus be very heavy indeed. This weight is made occasionally heavier by the fuzziness of some of the values by which social organization executives are presumed to be guided, and by the conflict among those values from which they are administratively pressured to choose. Conflict and controversy abound in the ethics of social work administration. The ethical lot of social organization executives can often be an unhappy one. Ethical choice, on the other hand, can be a stimulating challenge to executive ingenuity, not to mention executive conscience.

The Ethics of Organizational Decision-Making

What, among other things, may be especially time-consuming for executives, and for which they are likely to be held to account substantively and procedurally, is the way in which organization decisions are made and who participates in them. If business and industrial organizations share the concern about participation in organization decision-making, it is less on the basis of its morality than on the basis of its effectiveness in inducing acceptance of and cooperation with the decisions which are made. The assumption seems to be that decisions, especially decisions implying or leading to organizational innovations, are more effective when those who will be affected participate in them, and when those who may be relied upon for their implementation play a role in relation to them. In social organizations the premise for such participation—when clients and services to clients are involved, for example—is not simply its utility in the attainment of organization goals, but its morality: whatever participants may choose to do with their opportunities and their options in relation to their own fate, as inefficient as both they and the entire process of participation may be, their participation is "right" and just, and on that account alone merits administrative consideration and implementation. Staff and board, of course, are not as free, except in such instances as affect only them and their options. Executives have to consider, and provide for, the ultimate responsibilities of the organization. That, at least, is their ethical responsibility as monitors of the organization's purposes and functions.

All of this takes time. And it may not even work well. Perhaps that is why it is rarely done. But it would be ethical to do it since it represents organizational and administrative conduct and practice valued in its own right.

The Pain of Ethical Practice

It seems unrealistic to expect social organization executives to subject themselves to the kinds of dilatory and convoluted processes that administrative ethics often requires. It also seems unrealistic to expect social organization executives to make choices which defeat their own personal purposes, whether psychological, social, material, or emotional. But that is what ethics is primarily all about. Without the kinds of personal and organizational conflict—and occasional sacrifice—that such choices imply, there would not be very much to the ethics of social work administration. Such issues virtually demand a bit of agonizing if not outright personal pain and suffering.

Even if the subjective interests of executives are not the proximate cause of the conflict they may experience, they may still undergo stress when the choices they have to make concern concurrently operative moral obligations to multiple parties with unfortunately conflicting interests. In such cases, the issue in administrative ethics is not what is in the organization's own best institutional interests as against the interests of others. Nor is the issue that which is most practical as against administrative responsibility to the organization, to staff, or to others. The issue is often rather what is more or less equally owed by way of moral obligations to several parties with competing interests, most or all of which cannot practically be accommodated, and among which a priority of obligations must be ordered.

The pressure to make such choices is bound to result in great strain for social organization executives. But that, too, is in the nature of the ethics of social work administration. The evasion of such choices—perhaps because of the strain it generates—itself is apt to constitute unethical conduct, depending upon the nature of the choice to be made and the need for timely action in relation to it (cf. Levy, 1964). In short, the temptation to be unethical would intimidate Satan himself.

Affecting the Ethics of Others in the Social Organization

Although Hegarty and Sims studied ethical decision-making in business, the conditions that they discuss as provoking unethical conduct are relevant to ethical decision-making in social organizations, particularly when they emphasize the contagious effect of the behavior of executives and organizations:

> Mayer argues that there are three conditions that may provoke dishonest behavior: a) The individual may have an inclination toward dishonest behavior, b) the opportunity to engage in dishonest practices exists, and c) expected gains more than offset penalties. . . . If unethical decision making is rewarded, then higher incidence of unethical behavior is likely to occur. . . . The finding that threat of punishment has a counterbalance

influence has important implications for normative managerial practice. . . .

Unethical behavior also tended to increase when competitiveness was intensified. . . . When the emphasis is on the bottom line, it is not surprising that actions are taken in accordance with the rationalization asserting that the ends justify the means. . . .

If top management is to seriously deal with ethics, they must be willing to deal with the issue in a straightforward manner, specifying corporate policies and practices that will reinforce corporate members to maintain ethical guidelines. If there are no punishments associated with unethical behavior, and a competitive situation makes such behavior profitable, it is likely that individuals who are not endowed with high standards of ethical conduct by past training (of some kind) are likely to succumb to the temptation to reap the profits of unethical behavior by behaving unethically (1978, pp. 452, 456).

The responsibility of the social organization executive includes assistance in the development of the functional capacities of board and staff, and clients and members. As far as the ethics of social work administration is concerned, therefore, the responsibility of the executive includes the representation, the implementation, and the development of ethical practice in the social organization. And it includes the development of the capacity for ethical practice of everyone in the organization in relation to whom the executive has any administrative function to perform. It is incumbent upon the social organization executive to be ethical, and to inspire, encourage, and help others to become ethical, certainly in all of their operations and relationships in, and on behalf of, the organization.

This is a socialization function in that its aim is to generate an organizational culture which reflects, and is maximally conducive to, the valuation of a high standard of ethical conduct. And it is an educational function in that organization participants are helped to learn what ethics in social organizations consists of, the principles by which it is guided, and how it is done.

The leadership and management of a social organization are naturally critical means for representing the kind of behavior which is organizationally and administratively valued. The modeling of valued behavior is obviously a potent force in a social organization, especially in the emotionally charged relationships between the social organization executives and others. And such modeling is obviously an influential impetus to ethical conduct in the fulfillment of administrative responsibility. However, it is not sufficient or enduring enough. Imitation may be a high form of flattery, and may even represent conditioned ethical behavior which does have its utility for the administration of social organizations. But it is too limited and too unreliable for organizational and administrative purposes.

Education and Training for Ethical Practice

The objective which would more reliably guide the executive in the fulfillment of administrative responsibility in this connection is the identification and
reinforcement—in supervision and evaluation, for example, and in board and
staff meetings—of the kind of behavior which, it becomes gradually but forcefully evident, is the only kind of behavior that can be approved, sanctioned,
encouraged, and rewarded in the organization. In staff development programs
and collegial exchange, moreover, the reasons for selecting what is to be
valued in organizational conduct can be extensively and intensively explored so
that general principles of ethical practice, and the meaning of such codified
principles as already exist, can become increasingly serviceable and incorporated for independent application by staff members in their daily practice and
experience and perhaps in their own future practice as social organization
executives.

Whether directly or via delegation, it is the social organization executive's
administrative responsibility to provide staff members with opportunities to
learn to do their work better and better, and more and more ethically. It is also
the executive's job to see to it that improvement on both counts does not go
unrewarded in some way, but not without reflecting to staff members that
ethical as well as competent practice is fundamentally and significantly its own
highest reward.

The principles which guide the process of socialization and education for
ethical practice in staff in-service training apply also to the process of formal
education in schools in which organization personnel acquire the preparation
for the administrative functions they perform. For students who are learning to
be organization administrators, the opportunities for the acquisition of knowledge, skill, and attitudes for ethical administrative practice should be very
specifically and directly designed for that purpose. Where supervised field
practice is part of the school curriculum, as it is in social work education, the
ethical components and implications of students' practice experiences should be
thoroughly analyzed in classes and supervisory conferences. The objective
would be to identify issues in ethics, and principles and practices related to
them, so that students may learn to evaluate their own practice as well as the
practices of others. The objective would also be to arrive at general principles
of ethical administrative practice, and interpretations of existing principles as
found in organizational and professional codes. Approaches to the implementation of such principles can also be considered and compared.

It is obviously essential for teachers and supervisors to be informed about
the principles, and have conviction about them, and to be skilled in their
application. The application of principles of ethical administrative practice, it
must be emphasized, requires art and sensitivity as much as it does philosophical conviction. The way in which they are applied can be as unethical as the
failure to apply them.

For effective education for ethical administrative practice, every possible ethical issue in practice experience ought to be at least identified. As many issues as possible ought also to be explored in order to increase student sensitivity to the values which figure in each experience, in every relationship, and in every administrative intervention—and sensitivity to dministrators or not.

Administrative Ethics as Integral to Organizational Culture

There is much about the ethics of social work administration that everyone in social organizations ought to know. No service, program, or practice in any social organization exists in a social vacuum, or in an administrative vacuum, although there are times when it seems that way. Neither does any practitioner operate in a social or administrative vacuum, although some practitioners sometimes act as if they do. Administrative ethics, whatever its state and condition in a social organization, becomes and is an integral part of the organization culture. It constitutes as essential a part of the knowledge of organization participants as the structure, the policies, the procedures, the functions, and everything else that there is to know about the social organization.

Expanding and Developing the State of Administrative Ethics

Whatever the state and condition of the ethics of and in social organizations, there is in the ethics of social work administration invariably more depth and greater scope to be developed, to be known, and to be incorporated for occupational use. That at least should be the guiding motif in school curricula for those who contemplate careers and responsibility as social organization administrators, and for those who do not. It would not be amiss for students to be disquieted, and perhaps humble, about the reaches and implications of ethical responsibility in social organizations. There are values affecting human beings and human institutions that human service practitioners at all levels of social organization responsibility ought to feel an occupational responsibility to be committed to. Those values figure in all social organizations, regardless of their size, regardless of the variations in their purposes and structures. Commitment to these values and to their clarification and development, also represents, for career organization practitioners like social workers, commitment to act upon them and toward their realization, for the sake of organization clienteles and others, and for the commonweal. What these values are and should be, and what to do about them, are also lessons to be learned, not only by prospective social organization executives, but by all prospective social organization personnel.

Easy it is not, but necessary it is. Few social endeavors are more worthy of the effort.

REFERENCES

Hegarty, W. Harvey and Sims, Henry P., Jr. "Some Determinants of Unethical Decision Behavior: An Experiment," *Journal of Applied Psychology,* 63 (1978), 451-457.

Levy, Charles S. "The Classification of Personal Decisions: An Aid in Decision-Making," *Adult Leadership,* 13 (1964), 103-104, 127-128.

Levy, Charles S. *Education and Training for the Fundraising Function* (New York: The Lois and Samuel Silberman Fund for the Bureau for Careers in Jewish Service, 1973).

APPENDIX

Code of Ethics of the National Association of Social Workers

As adopted by the 1979 NASW Delegate Assembly, effective July 1, 1980.

National Association of Social Workers, Inc.
1425 H Street, N.W., Suite 600
Washington, D.C. 20005

Preamble

This code is intended to serve as a guide to the everyday conduct of members of the social work profession and as a basis for the adjudication of issues in ethics when the conduct of social workers is alleged to deviate from the standards expressed or implied in this code. It represents standards of ethical behavior for social workers in professional relationships with those served, with colleagues, with employers, with other individuals and professions, and with the community and society as a whole. It also embodies standards of ethical behavior governing individual conduct to the extent that such conduct is associated with an individual's status and identity as a social worker.

This code is based on the fundamental values of the social work profession that include the worth, dignity, and uniqueness of all persons as well as their rights and opportunities. It is also based on the nature of social work, which fosters conditions that promote these values.

In subscribing to and abiding by this code, the social worker is expected to view ethical responsibility in as inclusive a context as each situation demands and within which ethical judgement is required. The social worker is expected to take into consideration all the principles in this code that have a bearing upon any situation in which ethical judgement is to be exercised and professional intervention or conduct is planned. The course of action that the social worker chooses is expected to be consistent with the spirit as well as the letter of this code.

In itself, this code does not represent a set of rules that will prescribe all the behaviors of social workers in all the complexities of professional life. Rather, it offers general principles to guide conduct, and the judicious appraisal of conduct, in situations that have ethical implications. It provides the basis for making judgements about ethical actions before and after they occur. Frequently, the particular situation determines the ethical principles that apply and the manner of their application. In such cases, not only the particular ethical principles are taken into immediate consideration, but also the entire code and its spirit. Specific applications of ethical principles must be judged within the context in which they are being considered. Ethical behavior in a given situation must satisfy not only the judgement of the individual social worker, but also the judgement of an unbiased jury of professional peers.

This code should not be used as an instrument to deprive any social worker of the opportunity or freedom to practice with complete professional integrity; nor should any disciplinary action be taken on the basis of this code without maximum provision for safeguarding the rights of the social worker affected.

The ethical behavior of social workers results not from edict, but from a personal commitment of the individual. This code is offered to affirm the will and zeal of all social workers to be ethical and to act ethically in all that they do as social workers.

The following codified ethical principles should guide social workers in the various roles and relationships and at the various levels of responsibility in which they function professionally. These principles also serve as a basis for the adjudication by the National Association of Social Workers of issues in ethics.

In subscribing to this code, social workers are required to cooperate in its implementation and abide by any disciplinary rulings based on it. They should also take adequate measures to discourage, prevent, expose, and correct the unethical conduct of colleagues. Finally, social workers should be equally ready to defend and assist colleagues unjustly charged with unethical conduct.

National Association of Social Workers. Code of Ethics. Revised 1979, Published 1980.
Reprinted with permission of National Association of Social Workers, Inc.

Summary of Major Principles

I. The Social Worker's Conduct and Comportment as a Social Worker

A. **Propriety.**The Social worker should maintain high standards of personal conduct in the capacity or identity as social worker.

B. **Competence and Professional Development.** The social worker should strive to become and remain proficient in professional practice and the performance of professional functions.

C. **Service.** The social worker should regard as primary the service obligation of the social work profession.

D. **Integrity.** The social worker should act in accordance with the highest standards of professional integrity.

E. **Scholarship and Research.** The social worker engaged in study and research should be guided by the conventions of scholarly inquiry.

II. The Social Worker's Ethical Responsibility to Clients

F. **Primacy of Clients' Interests.** The social worker's primary responsibility is to clients.

G. **Rights and Prerogatives of Clients.** The social worker should make every effort to foster maximum self-determination on the part of clients.

H. **Confidentiality and Privacy.** The social worker should respect the privacy of clients and hold in confidence all information obtained in the course of professional service.

I. **Fees.** When setting fees, the social worker should ensure that they are fair, reasonable, considerate, and commensurate with the service performed and with due regard for the clients' ability to pay.

III. The Social Worker's Ethical Responsibility to Colleagues

J. **Respect, Fairness, and Courtesy.** The social worker should treat colleagues with respect, courtesy, fairness, and good faith.

K. **Dealing with Colleagues' Clients.** The social worker has the responsibility to relate to the clients of colleagues with full professional consideration.

IV. The Social Worker's Ethical Responsibility to Employers and Employing Organizations

L. **Commitments to Employing Organizations.** The social worker should adhere to commitments made to the employing organizations.

V. The Social Worker's Ethical Responsibility to the Social Work Profession

M. **Maintaining the Integrity of the Profession.** The social worker should uphold and advance the values, ethics, knowledge, and mission of the profession.

N. **Community Service.** The social worker should assist the profession in making social services available to the general public.

O. **Development of Knowledge.** The social worker should take responsibility for identifying, developing, and fully utilizing knowledge for professional practice.

VI. The Social Worker's Ethical Responsibility to Society

P. **Promoting the General Welfare.** The social worker should promote the general welfare of society.

The NASW Code of Ethics

I. The Social Worker's Conduct and Comportment as a Social Worker

A. Propriety—The Social worker should maintain high standards of personal conduct in the capacity or identity as social worker.

1. The private conduct of the social worker is a personal matter to the same degree as is any other person's, except when such conduct compromises the fulfillment of professional responsibilities.

2. The social worker should not participate in, condone, or be associated with dishonesty, fraud, deceit, or misrepresentation.

3. The social worker should distinguish clearly between statements and actions made as a private individual and as a representative of the social work profession or an organization or group.

B. Competence and Professional Development—The social worker should strive to become and remain proficient in professional practice and the performance of professional functions.

1. The social worker should accept responsibility or employment only on the basis of existing competence or the intention to acquire the necessary competence.

2. The social worker should not misrepresent professional qualifications, education, experience, or affiliations.

C. Service —The social worker should regard as primary the service obligation of the social work profession.

1. The social worker should retain ultimate responsibility for the quality and extent of the service that individual assumes, assigns, or performs.

2. The social worker should act to prevent practices that are inhumane or discriminatory against any person or group of persons.

D. Integrity —The social worker should act in accordance with the highest standards of professional integrity and impartiality.

1. The social worker should be alert to and resist the influences and pressures that interfere with the exercise of professional discretion and impartial judgement required for the performance of professional functions.

2. The social worker should not exploit professional relationships for personal gain.

E. **Scholarship and Research —The social worker engaged in study and research should be guided by the conventions of scholarly inquiry.**
1. The social worker engaged in research should consider carefully its possible consequences for human beings.
2. The social worker engaged in research should ascertain that the consent of participants in the research is voluntary and informed, without any implied deprivation or penalty for refusal to participate, and with due regard for participants' privacy and dignity.
3. The social worker engaged in research should protect participants from unwarranted physical or mental discomfort, distress, harm, danger, or deprivation.
4. The social worker who engages in the evaluation of services or cases should discuss them only for the professional purposes and only with persons directly and professionally concerned with them.
5. Information obtained about participants in research should be treated as confidential.
6. The social worker should take credit only for work actually done in connection with scholarly and research endeavors and credit contributions made by others.

II. The Social Worker's Ethical Responsibility to Clients

F. **Primacy of Clients' Interests—The social worker's primary responsibility is to clients.**
1. The social worker should serve clients with devotion, loyalty, determination, and the maximum application of professional skill and competence.
2. The social worker should not exploit relationships with clients for personal advantage, or solicit the clients of one's agency for private practice.
3. The social worker should not practice, condone, facilitate or collaborate with any form of discrimination on the basis of race, color, sex, sexual orientation, age, religion, national origin, marital status, political belief, mental or physical handicap, or any other preference or personal characteristic, condition or status.
4. The social worker should avoid relationships or commitments that conflict with the interests of clients.
5. The social worker should under no circumstances engage in sexual activities with clients.
6. The social worker should provide clients with accurate and complete information regarding the extent and nature of the services available to them.
7. The social worker should apprise clients of their risks, rights, opportunities, and obligations associated with social service to them.
8. The social worker should seek advice and counsel of colleagues and supervisors whenever such consultation is in the best interest of clients.
9. The social worker should terminate service to clients, and professional relationships with them, when such service and relationships

are no longer required or no longer serve the clients' needs or interests.
10. The social worker should withdraw services precipitously only under unusual circumstances, giving careful consideration to all factors in the situation and taking care to minimize possible adverse effects.
11. The social worker who anticipates the termination or interruption of service to clients should notify clients promptly and seek the transfer, referral, or continuation of service in relation to the clients' needs and preferences.

G. **Rights and Prerogatives of Clients-The social worker should make every effort to foster maximum self-determination on the part of clients.**
1. When the social worker must act on behalf of a client who has been adjudged legally incompetent, the social worker should safeguard the interests and rights of that client.
2. When another individual has been legally authorized to act in behalf of a client, the social worker should deal with that person always with the client's best interest in mind.
3. The social worker should not engage in any action that violates or diminishes the civil or legal rights of clients.

H. **Confidentiality and Privacy —The social worker should respect the privacy of clients and hold in confidence all information obtained in the course of professional service.**
1. The social worker should share with others confidences revealed by clients, without their consent, only for **compelling professional reasons.**
2. The social worker should inform clients fully about the limits of confidentiality in a given situation, the purposes for which information is obtained, and how it may be used.
3. The social worker should afford clients reasonable access to any official social work records concerning them.
4. When providing clients with access to records, the social worker should take due care to protect the confidences of others contained in those records.
5. The social worker should obtain informed consent of clients before taping, recording, or permitting third party observation of their activities.

I. **Fees —When setting fees, the social worker should ensure that they are fair, reasonable, considerate, and commensurate with the service performed and with due regard for the clients' ability to pay.**
1. The social worker should not divide a fee or accept or give anything of value for receiving or making a referral.

III. The Social Worker's Ethical Responsibility to Colleagues

J. **Respect, Fairness, and Courtesy —The social worker should treat colleagues with respect courtesy, fairness, and good faith.**
1. The social worker should cooperate with colleagues to promote professional interests and concerns.

2. The social worker should respect confidences shared by colleagues in the course of their professional relationships and transactions.

3. The social worker should create and maintain conditions of practice that facilitate ethical and competent professional performance by colleagues.

4. The social worker should treat with respect, and represent accurately and fairly, the qualifications, views, and findings of colleagues and use appropriate channels to express judgements on these matters.

5. The social worker who replaces or is replaced by a colleague in professional practice should act with consideration for the interest, character, and reputation of that colleague.

6. The social worker should not exploit a dispute between a colleague and employers to obtain a position or otherwise advance the social worker's interest.

7. The social worker should seek arbitration or mediation when conflicts with colleagues require resolution for compelling professional reasons.

8. The social worker should extend to colleagues of other professions the same respect and cooperation that is extended to social work colleagues.

9. The social worker who serves as an employer, supervisor, or mentor to colleagues should make orderly and explicit arrangements regarding the conditions of their continuing professional relationship.

10. The social worker who has the responsibility for employing and evaluating the performance of other staff members, should fulfill such responsibility in a fair, considerate, and equitable manner, on the basis of clearly enunciated criteria.

11. The social worker who has the responsibility for evaluating the performance of employees, supervisees, or students should share evaluations with them.

K. Dealing with Colleagues' Clients —The social worker has the responsibility to relate to the clients of colleagues with full professional consideration.

1. The social worker should not solicit the clients of colleagues.

2. The social worker should not assume professional responsibility for the clients of another agency or a colleague without appropriate communication with that agency or colleague.

3. The social worker who serves the clients of colleagues, during a temporary absence or emergency, should serve those clients with the same consideration as that afforded any client.

IV. The Social Worker's Ethical Responsibility to Employers and Employing Organizations

L. Commitments to Employing Organization ——The social worker should adhere to commitments made to the employing organization.

1. The social worker should work to improve the employing agency's policies and procedures, and the efficiency and effectiveness of its services.

2. The social worker should not accept employment or arrange student field placements in an organization which is currently under

public sanction by NASW for violating personnel standards, or imposing limitations on or penalties for professional actions on behalf of clients.

3. The social worker should act to prevent and eliminate discrimination in the employing organization's work assignments and in its employment policies and practices.

4. The social worker should use with scrupulous regard, and only for the purpose for which they are intended, the resources of the employing organization.

V. The Social Worker's Ethical Responsibility to the Social Work Profession

M. Maintaining the Integrity of the Profession—The social worker should uphold and advance the values, ethics, knowledge, and mission of the profession.

1. The social worker should protect and enhance the dignity and integrity of the profession and should be responsible and vigorous in discussion and criticism of the profession.

2. The social worker should take action through appropriate channels against unethical conduct by any other member of the profession.

3. The social worker should act to prevent the unauthorized and unqualified practice of social work.

4. The social worker should make no misrepresentation in advertising as to qualifications, competence, service, or results to be achieved.

N. Community Service—The social worker should assist the profession in making social services available to the general public.

1. The social worker should contribute time and professional expertise to activities that promote respect for the utility, the integrity, and the competence of the social work profession.

2. The social worker should support the formulation, development, enactment and implementation of social policies of concern to the profession.

O. Development of Knowledge—The social worker should take responsibility for identifying, developing, and fully utilizing knowledge for professional practice.

1. The social worker should base practice upon recognized knowledge relevant to social work.

2. The social worker should critically examine, and keep current with emerging knowledge relevant to social work.

3. The social worker should contribute to the knowledge base of social work and share research knowledge and practice wisdom with colleagues.

VI. The Social Worker's Ethical Responsibility to Society

P. Promoting the General Welfare—The social worker should promote the general welfare of society.

1. The social worker should act to prevent and eliminate discrimination against any person or group on the basis of race, color, sex, sexual orientation, age, religion, national origin, marital status, political belief, mental or physical handicap, or any other preference or personal characteristic, condition, or status.

2. The social worker should act to ensure that all persons have access to the resources, services, and opportunities which they require.
3. The social worker should act to expand choice and opportunity for all persons, with special regard for disadvantaged or oppressed groups and persons.
4. The social worker should promote conditions that encourage respect for the diversity of cultures which constitute American society.
5. The social worker should provide appropriate professional services in public emergencies.
6. The social worker should advocate changes in policy and legislation to improve social conditions and to promote social justice.
7. The social worker should encourage informed participation by the public in shaping social policies and institutions.

INDEX